DATE

Confidentiality Versus the Duty to Protect: Foreseeable Harm in the Practice of Psychiatry

ISSUES IN
PSYCHIATRY

Joseph Bloom, M.D.
Series Editor

Confidentiality Versus the Duty to Protect: Foreseeable Harm in the Practice of Psychiatry

Edited by

"Ed."

James C. Beck, M.D., Ph.D.

Associate Professor of Psychiatry, Harvard Medical School; and Director, Cambridge Court Clinic, Cambridge, Massachusetts

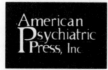

American Psychiatric Press, Inc.

Washington, DC
London, England

Copyright © 1990 American Psychiatric Press, Inc.
ALL RIGHTS RESERVED
Manufactured in the United States of America
93 92 91 90 4 3 2 1
First Edition

American Psychiatric Press, Inc.
1400 K Street, N.W., Washington, D.C. 20005

The paper used in this publication meets the minimum requirements of the American National Standard for Information Sciences—Permanence of Paper for Printed Library Materials, ANSI Z39.48-1984.   ∞

Library of Congress Cataloging-in-Publication Data

Confidentiality versus the duty to protect: foreseeable harm in the practice
   of psychiatry / edited by James C. Beck. — 1st ed.
      p.   cm. — (Issues in psychiatry)
   ISBN 0-88048-170-6 (alk. paper)
   1. Psychotherapist and patient—Moral and ethical aspects.
   2. Confidential communications—Physicians. 3. Patient advocacy—Moral and ethical aspects. I. Beck, James C., 1934–   .
   II. Series.
   [DNLM: 1. Confidentiality. 2. Ethics, Medical. 3. Forensic
   Psychiatry. 4. Patient Advocacy.   W 740 C748]
   RC480.8.C66   1990
   616.89′0232—dc20
   DNLM/DLC
   for Library of Congress   90-13
                                                                    CIP

British Library Cataloguing in Publication Data

A CIP record is available from the British Library.

For Susan

Contents

Contributors

Kenneth Appelbaum, M.D.
Assistant Professor of Psychiatry, University of Massachusetts Medical School, Worcester; and Director of Forensic Service, Worcester State Hospital, Worcester, Massachusetts

Paul S. Appelbaum, M.D.
A.F. Zeleznik Professor of Psychiatry and Director, Program in Psychiatry and Law, University of Massachusetts Medical School, Worcester, Massachusetts

Richard Barnum, M.D.
Clinical Instructor in Psychiatry, Harvard Medical School, Cambridge; Assistant in Psychiatry, Children's Hospital, Boston; and Director, Boston Juvenile Court Clinic, Boston, Massachusetts

Stephen J. Bartels, M.D.
Research Associate, New Hampshire–Dartmouth Psychiatric Research Center; and Assistant Professor of Clinical Psychiatry, Dartmouth Medical School, Hanover, New Hampshire

James C. Beck, M.D., Ph.D.
Associate Professor of Psychiatry, Harvard Medical School; and Director, Cambridge Court Clinic, Cambridge, Massachusetts

Joseph D. Bloom, M.D.
Professor of Psychiatry and Chairman of the Department of
Psychiatry, School of Medicine, Oregon Health Sciences
University, Portland, Oregon

Robert E. Drake, M.D., Ph.D.
Director, New Hampshire–Dartmouth Psychiatric Research
Center; and Associate Professor of Psychiatry, Dartmouth
Medical School, Hanover, New Hampshire

David J. Drummond, Ph.D.
Assistant Professor of Medical Psychology, Psychology
Service, Veterans Administration Medical Center; and the
Department of Medical Psychology, School of Medicine,
Oregon Health Sciences University, Portland Oregon

Spencer Eth, M.D.
Assistant Professor of Psychiatry, University of California,
Los Angeles, School of Medicine; Clinical Associate Professor
of Psychiatry, University of Southern California School of
Medicine, Los Angeles; and Acting Chief, Psychiatry Service,
Brentwood Division, West Los Angeles Veterans
Administration Medical Center, Los Angeles, California

Bruce C. Gage, M.D.
Staff Psychiatrist, Sepulveda Veterans Administration Medical
Center; and Assistant Clinical Professor of Psychiatry,
University of California, Los Angeles, School of Medicine,
Los Angeles, California

Sally L. Godard, M.D.
Adjunct Assistant Professor of Psychiatry, Department of
Psychiatry, School of Medicine, Oregon Health Sciences
University; and Director of Psychiatric Education, Oregon
Mental Health Division, Portland, Oregon

Joseph B. Layde, M.D., J.D.
Director of Forensic Unit, Milwaukee County Mental Health
Complex; Forensic Psychiatric Consultant, Milwaukee
Psychiatric Hospital; and Assistant Professor, Department of
Psychiatry and Mental Health Sciences, Medical College of
Wisconsin, Milwaukee, Wisconsin

Gregory B. Leong, M.D.
Assistant Professor of Psychiatry, University of California,
Los Angeles, School of Medicine; and Staff Psychiatrist,
Brentwood Division, West Los Angeles Veterans
Administration Medical Center, Los Angeles, California

Robert I. Simon, M.D.
Clinical Professor of Psychiatry and Director, Program in
Psychiatry and Law, Georgetown University, School of
Medicine, Washington, DC

Landy F. Sparr, M.D., M.A.
Associate Professor of Psychiatry, Psychiatry Service,
Veterans Administration Medical Center; and the Department
of Psychiatry, School of Medicine, Oregon Health Sciences
University, Portland, Oregon

Kimberly A. White, M.D.
Assistant Director of Psychiatric Emergency Services,
Cambridge Hospital; and Instructor in Psychiatry, Harvard
Medical School, Cambridge, Massachusetts

CHAPTER ONE

The Basic Issues

James C. Beck, M.D., Ph.D.

Confidentiality has long been a cornerstone of the practice of medicine and psychiatry. Hippocrates wrote:

> Whatsoever things I shall see or hear concerning the life of men, in my attendance on the sick or even apart therefrom, which ought not to be noised abroad, I will keep silence thereon, counting such things to be as holy secrets. (1)

Slovenko points out that Hippocrates' use of the word *ought* suggests some element of judgment about the limits on confidentiality. The ban on "noising about" is not absolute.

Skipping forward 2,500 years, the Code of Ethics for Psychiatrists states:

> A physician shall . . . safeguard patient confidences within the constraints of the law. . . . Confidentiality is essential to psychiatric treatment. . . . Because of the sensitive and private nature of the information with which the psychiatrist deals, he/she must be circumspect in the information that he/she chooses to disclose to others about a patient. . . . A psychiatrist may release confidential information only with the authorization of the patient or under proper legal compulsion. (2, p. 5)

Exceptions to Confidentiality

Until the past few years, there were few generally recognized exceptions to the rule that the psychiatrist should preserve the patient's confidentiality. If a patient required civil commitment, psychiatrists provided the necessary information to the receiving hospital without the patient's permission. Members of an inpatient treatment team would share clinical information without obtaining the patient's permission. In either case, the psychiatrist breached confidentiality primarily in the patient's interest, not in the interest of someone else.

Within general medicine, the law required physicians to report persons with epilepsy operating machinery, persons with dangerous or contagious diseases, and persons with gunshot or knife wounds. These reports served primarily to protect the public. Although psychiatrists were subject to them, these exceptions had few effects on the practice of psychiatry and none on other psychotherapeutic professions.

In the past 20 years there has been a dramatic increase in the number and type of exceptions to confidentiality. Unlike the earlier breaches, these exceptions are not mandated for the benefit of the patient. Psychotherapists are required to report information to third-party payers as a condition of payment. Another exception is the psychotherapist's *Tarasoff* duty to protect third parties who are foreseeably endangered by their patients. A third exception, mandated by law in all 50 states, is reporting of child abuse. Many jurisdictions now have statutes mandating report of elder abuse as well.

There are numerous other statutory exceptions to confidentiality as well. In Massachusetts they are

1. When the psychotherapist determines that the patient requires hospitalization
2. In any proceeding, except one involving child custody, in which the patient introduces his or her mental or emotional condition as an element of the case, and the judge finds that the therapist should disclose
3. In the event that a patient dies and his or her will is contested, and mental state was an issue
4. In child custody cases when the judge thinks it is necessary to preserve the child's best interests
5. If the patient sues the therapist

Other Massachusetts law holds that social workers (but not other mental health professionals) may disclose patient communications about the contemplation or commission of a crime. And finally, the director of any Department of Mental Health facility is required to report to the district attorney knowledge of any felony committed by a person under the care of that facility.

The Tarasoff Exception

The original *Tarasoff* case involved a man disappointed by love who became depressed and entered psychotherapy. He told his therapist that he was thinking of killing the woman involved, and some months later he carried out his threat.

Her survivors sued, and in 1974 the California Supreme Court said the therapist owed a duty to the victim based on the fact that the therapist had a therapist-patient relationship with the man who killed her.

> When a doctor or psychotherapist, in the exercise of his professional skill and knowledge, determines or should determine, that a warning is essential to avert danger arising from the medical or psychological condition of his patient, he incurs a legal obligation to give that warning. (3, p. 914)

Therefore, the duty to warn became one of the responsibilities of the psychotherapist. In 1976, the California Supreme Court reheard the *Tarasoff* case, and issued a second opinion.

> When a therapist determines or pursuant to the standard of his profession should determine, that his patient presents a serious danger of violence to another, he incurs an obligation to use reasonable care to protect the intended victim against such danger. The discharge of this duty may require the therapist to take one or more of various steps depending upon the nature of the case. Thus, it may call for him to warn the intended victim or others likely to apprise the intended victim of danger, to notify the police, or take whatever steps are reasonably necessary under the circumstances. (4, p. 346)

The change in language from the first to the second opinion illustrates the increasing complexity of the therapist's responsibility. In 1974, the court made a relatively clear and limited directive: warn the victim. In 1976, the court instructed the therapist to use professional judgment, and so greatly expanded the psychotherapist's possible choices of action.

Since *Tarasoff* there have been over 70 published legal cases in which psychiatrists and other psychotherapists as well as hospitals and other health care facilities have been named as defendants in suits alleging breach of the duty to protect. The facts in these cases have at times differed rather dramatically from those in the original *Tarasoff* case.

Tarasoff involved a specific threat to a named victim. Since then, courts have found a duty to protect when a patient

1. Drove his car recklessly and killed another driver (5)
2. Shot up a nightclub and injured random strangers (6)
3. Drove her car into a tree, killing herself and seriously injuring her daughter (7)
4. Killed a woman whom he never threatened (8)
5. Burned a barn after he threatened to do so (9)

And there are others.

The Present Climate

Clearly, the courts have expanded the therapist's duty to protect. In earlier times, psychotherapists were expected to listen to their patients and try to understand and help them. A therapist's duty was to the patient, and essentially only to the patient. Therapists helped society only indirectly by helping their patients to become better-functioning members of that society. Now it is not enough for therapists to treat their patients. The courts have made it clear that therapists are expected to exercise their professional judgment to prevent their patients from causing foreseeable harm to others.

The result of this expanded duty has been to increase substantially the range of potential threats that psychotherapists must consider. The specter of acquired immunodeficiency syndrome (AIDS)–related *Tarasoff* suits troubles many psychiatrists. Are sexual partners of persons with AIDS foreseeably endangered? Of course they are. Does this create a legal duty for the psychotherapist of an AIDS patient? And if it does create a duty, how does the therapist fulfill it?

Suppose a patient tells her therapist that her prior therapist and she had sexual relations. Suppose the therapist hears that this same therapist has had sexual relations with other patients. What is the therapist's duty? Does he or she have a duty to reveal this communication? and if so, to whom? with the patient's permission? or without?

Many psychiatrists are aware of these problems. A smaller number have confronted one or more of them in practice. Many psychiatrists are troubled about how to deal with the potential conflict between the duty to maintain a patient's confidentiality and the duty to prevent foreseeable harm.

The exceptions to confidentiality have multiplied, and the possible ways to deal with the exceptions have increased in number and complexity. The profession may be in danger of forgetting that these are exceptions. What occurs is a kind of figure-ground reversal. When there are too many exceptions, the exceptions become prominent, and the rule fades into the background.

Confidentiality and Privilege

Almost all psychiatrists know and understand the basic duty to preserve confidentiality. There is some confusion, however, about confidentiality and privilege. Privilege is a legal term, and it is applicable only in legal proceedings. It refers to who has the legal right to release or withhold information. At least 49 states have laws stating that information about patients is privileged, although the law of privilege varies from state to state.

Privilege lies with the patient, not with the psychiatrist. This means that, unless ordered to do so by a court, a psychiatrist cannot release information about a patient without the patient's permission. It also means that the patient can order the psychiatrist to release information and the psychiatrist is obligated to do so, unless the psychiatrist can claim some privilege of his or her own, for example, protection under the Fifth Amendment.

Practical Hints

In a legal proceeding, control of information about the patient rests with the patient, not with the psychiatrist. This is true for release of records as well as oral testimony. Many psychiatrists erroneously believe that they have control over when and to whom their records may be released. They are wrong. In a legal proceeding the patient has the right and authority to decide about release of clinical information. There are exceptions to this (see below) when a judge may order release of clinical information, but the choice in a legal proceeding is not the clinician's.

Subpoena is another subject of confusion. Subpoena refers to an order, as part of a legal proceeding, to produce something or someone. This means that the person or thing subpoenaed must be at the court available for examination at the time specified by the subpoena. Attorneys may tell you that you must turn over documents to them pursuant to a subpoena. That is never true. You must make them available to a court, which can then decide whether to turn them over to the party who subpoenaed them.

As a general rule, if you are involved in an adversary proceeding or you have a patient who is involved in an adversary proceeding, do not take the adversary attorney's word for anything. Always check with the attorney for your side before saying or doing anything. For example, if you are subpoenaed, the attorney acting for you or your patient may move to quash the subpoena. If this motion is successful, you do not have to appear.

No matter how official the piece of paper looks or how insistent the attorney may be, never do what he or she says unless your side's attorney agrees. Remember, only a judge can order you to do anything.

This book is designed to help psychiatrists and other psychotherapists deal with the problems created by the exceptions to confidentiality. The mental health professional must now have some knowledge of relevant law. Without such knowledge, the clinician carries the double burden of ignorance and anxiety. The wish to lighten that burden is the motive for this book.

This book is written by clinicians for clinicians. In it we present a discussion of law as it relates to the clinical issues of confidentiality versus the duty to protect. If a clinician knows and understands the law, he or she can practice with legal concerns receding into the background of consciousness. Attention can focus on the patient and the clinical issues, which is where it belongs.

Plan of the Book

This book is divided broadly into two sections. In the first section we present this chapter on basic issues, an overview of the law, and chapters on applications of the law in specific clinical settings. There are chapters addressing clinical practice in private office practice, in the emergency room, and in the hospital.

In the chapter on private practice we present several case examples, each with detailed discussion of evaluation and treatment issues. This discussion is applicable to practice in any setting. For this reason, Chapter 3 is recommended to every reader, not just the private practitioner.

In the second section we present chapters on specific clinical situations in which the duty to protect arises. There are chapters on issues relating to children and families, on sexual misconduct of therapists, on HIV-positive patients, on patients with dual diagnoses of mental disorder and substance abuse, and on two other problematic diagnoses: antisocial personality and posttraumatic stress disorder. There is also a chapter on what happens when a state requires psychiatrists to assess whether their patients are safe to drive. In the final chapter we present a clinical case in which the patient posed a unique threat to the potential victim. This case involved clinical and forensic problems that were initially vexing, but were ultimately resolved successfully.

References

1. Hippocrates: Oath, quoted by Slovenko R, in Kaplan HI, Sadock BJ (eds): Comprehensive Textbook of Psychiatry. Baltimore, MD, Williams & Wilkins, 1980, p 1988
2. American Psychiatric Association: Principles of Medical Ethics With Annotations Especially Applicable to Psychiatry. Washington, DC, American Psychiatric Association, 1986
3. Tarasoff v Regents of the University of California, 529 P2d 553, 118 Cal Rptr 129 (Cal Sup Ct 1974)
4. Tarasoff v Regents of the University of California, 551 P2d 334, 17 Cal3d 425 (Cal Sup Ct 1976)

5. Naidu v Laird, 539 A2d 1064 (Del Sup Ct 1988)
6. Lipari v Sears, 497 FSupp 185 (D Neb 1980)
7. Schuster v Altenberg, 424 NW2d 159, 87-0115 (Wisc Sup Ct 1988)
8. Jablonski v U.S., 712 F2d 391 (9th Cir 1983)
9. Peck v The Counseling Service of Addison County, 499 A2d 422 (Vt 1985)

CHAPTER TWO

Current Status of the Duty to Protect

James C. Beck, M.D., Ph.D.

Since *Tarasoff*, many courts have held that psychotherapists have a duty to protect the public as well as a duty to maintain patient confidentiality. The duty to protect arises whenever a therapist becomes aware that a patient's probable future behavior suggests a threat of foreseeable harm.

Plaintiffs bring *Tarasoff* suits after a patient has seriously injured or killed a third party. The plaintiff claims that the injury resulted from the therapist's breach of the duty to protect the victim from foreseeable harm. In deciding these cases, the court must first determine whether as a matter of law there was a duty to protect. Only if the court decides that there was such a duty does it reach the issue of whether the defendant's conduct breached the duty.

Although the duty to protect dramatically expands the potential liability of psychotherapists, the number of *Tarasoff* suits remains surprisingly small, and only a few psychiatrists have been found liable for breach of the *Tarasoff* duty. There have been just four published cases in which defendants have been found liable for breach of a *Tarasoff* duty (1–4). Two of these defendants were state hospital psychiatrists (3,4), one was a Veterans Administration (VA) psychiatrist (1), and one was a counselor in a community clinic (2).

Estimates of unpublished cases are necessarily imprecise. The following analysis draws on published statistics on number of malpractice suits and on estimates of knowledgeable attorneys. Approximately 50 psychiatrists each year are sued for breach of the duty to protect. Roughly two-thirds of these cases settle before trial. Of the trials, roughly two-thirds result in verdicts for the defendant. This analysis generates an estimate of 17 trials a year, and 6 psychiatrists a year found liable. The American Psychiatric

Association (APA) now has over 35,000 members. Odds on an APA member being sued for breach of the duty to protect, going to trial, and being found liable are 5,800 to 1 in any one year.

Courts have held that there is a duty to protect when the violence is foreseeable and the therapist has sufficient control over the patient's behavior to prevent the violence. Three factors contribute to a determination of foreseeability: 1) a history of violence, 2) a threat to a named or clearly identifiable victim, and 3) a plausible motive. If two or more of these are present, the courts usually find that violence was foreseeable. If only one is present, the courts sometimes do and sometimes do not find foreseeable violence. If none is present, courts rarely find that violence was foreseeable.

Courts assess control in part based on whether the case involves an outpatient or the release of an inpatient. In cases involving release of hospitalized patients, the courts usually find that sufficient control is present. By contrast, courts find a duty to control in about one-half of outpatient cases, and in one-half they do not find a duty to control.

There have been a few questionable decisions in which courts have held therapists accountable for future violence without adequate basis. However, contrary to the fears of many therapists, courts have rarely held therapists liable merely for failing to predict violence. In almost all cases, if a patient has been violent and the therapist has conformed to usual professional standards, courts have declined to find liability.

The following selected group of cases includes the general trends in duty to protect case law and specific holdings of particular interest. In the latter category are three cases: one favorable to psychiatry (5), one unfavorable (3), and one initially unfavorable at the appellate level (15); however, when this latter case was remanded for trial, the defendant was found not to be negligent.

Recent Case Law

Limitations of the Duty to Protect

Inpatient release cases.   In *Canon v. Thumudo* (5), the Michigan Supreme Court reversed finally the original finding of liability in *Davis v. Lhim* (4). *Davis* is one of two or three *Tarasoff* cases that most troubled psychiatrists.

In *Davis*, a voluntary state hospital patient was discharged at his own request. Two months after discharge, he became difficult to manage, and relatives sent him to live with his mother. He killed her during a struggle in which she tried to take a shotgun away from him.

The patient had no history of violence, he had questionably threatened his mother once 2 years earlier, and there was no known motive. Nor was there any allegation that the doctor had failed to use due care in discharging him. A jury awarded $500,000 to her survivors.

There were several appeals, and each time the court upheld the original verdict. One issue the appeals court considered is whether a state hospital doctor is immune from suit. Before *Canon*, the Michigan Supreme Court distinguished discretionary activities, which are immune, from ministerial actions, which are not immune. Discretionary activities are those in which the person exercises independent judgment. Ministerial activities are those in which the individual follows policy so that little or no independent judgment is required.

In *Canon*, the Michigan Supreme Court held that Dr. Lhim's professional actions were discretionary and therefore immune. On this basis, 13 years after the patient killed his mother, the courts finally overturned the original verdict. Although the legal reasoning is tortured, the final result is consistent with mainstream legal opinion. Other courts have refused to find a duty to protect in the absence of a history of violence, clear threat, and plausible motive.

In *Novak v. Rathnam* (6), an Illinois court held that *Tarasoff* applies only when a patient threatens an identified victim. The court limited the duty, holding that it would not extend to victims who are not readily identifiable.

In *Novak*, a paranoid schizophrenic man who refused antipsychotic medication was involuntarily hospitalized after exhibiting hostile and threatening behavior. In the hospital, he refused medication and psychosocial treatment, and he was released after 6 weeks. Fourteen months later, he committed an armed robbery in Florida, during which he shot and killed the victim. Her survivors sued.

The court held as a matter of law that a discharge 14 months earlier could not be the proximate cause of an injury. Because the patient had never threatened the victim, the violence was not foreseeable and there was no duty to protect. The appeals court upheld the trial court's dismissal of the suit.

In *Phillips v. Roy* (7), a Louisiana court held that a complaint based on patient violence 19 months after discharge did not state a cause of action. The hospital had discharged the patient appropriately, and he had apparently done well for 19 months. However, 15 months after discharge, the man stopped outpatient treatment and antipsychotic medication. Nineteen months after discharge, the ex-patient went on a rampage, shooting black people at random, and he killed the plaintiff's decedent.

Psychiatrists have wondered whether they are liable for violence of discharged patients into the indefinite future. These two cases appear to set some limits on potential liability based solely on the passage of time.

Outpatient cases.   *Cooke v. Berlin* (8) is the first *Tarasoff* case to reach the appeals court in Arizona. The trial court had granted summary judgment for the defendant, that is, had dismissed the case finding no basis for a suit. The appeals court affirmed this judgment, holding that the psychiatrist-patient relationship was not sufficient in and of itself to give rise to a duty on the part of a psychiatrist to control a patient who murdered a third party.

In February 1982, in Arizona, a 22-year-old woman began therapy with a social worker after deciding she was under surveillance by the CIA. The social worker diagnosed paranoia. A psychiatrist agreed and prescribed antipsychotics. The patient later developed the belief that a local disc jockey was spying on her through her radio.

In June 1982, the woman broke off contact with the treating agency and went to Virginia. There she concluded that the only way to end the spying was to kill the disc jockey. She did not tell anyone about this decision. In August, she returned to Arizona, stole a gun, and fatally shot the disc jockey.

The plaintiff's expert claimed the system was negligent in having a social worker do the work of a physician, and that the doctor was negligent in failing to correct a faulty diagnosis. The court concluded that this raised an issue of fact sufficient to avoid summary judgment for the defendant. Having drawn the conclusion that the defendant could have been negligent in diagnosis and treatment of the patient, the court then went on to consider whether this negligence gave rise to any liability for the victim's death.

The plaintiffs argued that there was liability. They argued following *Lipari v. Sears* (9) and *Petersen v. Washington* (10) that the psychiatrist-patient relationship in and of itself was sufficient to create a duty to control. The court declined to accept this, saying, "In our opinion, the majority and better reasoned cases . . . have concluded that the duty to control should not be imposed solely because of that relationship" (8, p. 835). The court found that the plaintiff's claim of negligence was based on a theory of duty that it rejected. Therefore, the court upheld summary judgment for the defendant.

Bardoni v. Kim (11) involved a paranoid schizophrenic patient who shot and killed his mother and brother. The patient had no history of violence, or of threatening his mother. Therefore, the court held that the psychiatrist had no duty to protect the mother.

The patient had threatened his brother, and he believed his brother was plotting against him and had given him a hernia. The patient had told this to workers at a psychiatric facility in another state. Family members knew this but did not tell the psychiatrist.

The court found that there was a duty to protect the brother on the ground that the psychiatrist could have found out about this threat if he had sent for the patient's records.

The court limited the duty to "readily identifiable" victims, while holding the psychiatrist responsible for knowing what was in the patient's old records. This is the fourth published case (1,2,4,11) in which courts have held psychiatrists responsible for reviewing old records.

Several Michigan courts have declined to find a duty to protect in the absence of a psychotherapeutic relationship. In *Paul v. Plymouth General Hospital* (12) the court held that a general hospital emergency room physician had no duty to warn. A woman attempted suicide after difficulties with her boyfriend. A general physician treated her in the emergency room after her attempt and throughout her subsequent hospital stay, during which the patient refused psychiatric consultation. Eleven days after being discharged, the patient shot and killed her boyfriend and herself.

The court found no duty to hospitalize the patient based on her refusal to see a psychiatrist. The doctor had no duty to warn because there was no special relationship between doctor and patient as it related to the patient's mental or emotional condition. The doctor had no way to discover the patient's dangerous potential because the patient refused to see a psychiatrist. Finally, the court noted that, even if there were a duty to warn, it was not the proximate cause of the boyfriend's death because he already knew the patient was a danger to him.

This court clearly accepted the argument that psychiatrists are uniquely capable of assessing dangerousness. That could prove to be a double-edged sword in future cases.

In *Hinkelman v. Borgess Medical Center* (13), a paranoid man threatened his girlfriend. She moved out, but brought him to a psychiatric hospital. He signed in, but had second thoughts. He then began choking his girlfriend while they were in a conference room. Security came and rescued her and she left. The patient signed out against medical advice and signed in again the following day. The girlfriend pressed charges.

Nine days later, the patient raped his former girlfriend. Two weeks after that, while out on bail, he kidnapped her and shot and killed a security guard, his former girlfriend, and himself.

The court held that there was no special relationship between the hospital and the patient because he was not in the hospital long enough to be evaluated, the hospital had no duty to keep the patient in the hospital, and the hospital had no duty to seek the patient's commitment.

Violence, in this case, appears to have been foreseeable. There was a history of violence, a clearly indentifiable victim, and a motive. Nevertheless, the court found no duty. This is one of several Michigan cases in which the courts limit the *Tarasoff* duty. Michigan courts appear to be limiting the duty either to cases in which there is a psychotherapist-patient relationship as distinct from a doctor-patient relationship, or to cases in which a hospital has a meaningful clinical relationship rather than merely a brief or clinically insignificant one.

Duty to Protect Is Present

Inpatient release cases. In *Pangborn v. Saad* (14), a North Carolina court entered judgment in favor of the staff psychiatrist, and the plaintiff appealed. The appeals court found that the plaintiff did state a cause of action against the physician who released the plaintiff's brother from the state hospital. Less than 16 hours after discharge, the patient allegedly stabbed his sister 20 times with a butcher knife.

The patient had a history of psychiatric treatment beginning in childhood and had previously attacked a family member. He had been involuntarily hospitalized seven times and had threatened his family shortly before his discharge. On the day of the patient's release, the family met with the doctor and said they feared the patient. They asked that he not be released.

The court said the plaintiff's complaint stated "a claim for actionable negligence, namely that the defendant breached a duty that he owed to the plaintiff" (14, p. 367), but the court did not specify what the duty was. The court remanded the case for trial. To my knowledge, it has not yet been decided.

Naidu v. Laird (3) resulted in a finding of gross negligence against the doctor and an award of $1.4 million to the plaintiff. *Naidu* has excited considerable adverse comment from psychiatrists. However, the summaries published in the psychiatric press have not included the extensive prior history. The history is important in forming an opinion about the verdict.

The case involved a former state hospital patient who caused a fatal auto accident. The patient, who had an extensive psychiatric history, was diagnosed with severe chronic paranoid schizophrenia in 1959 and was hospitalized 19 times between 1962 and 1977. He repeatedly refused antipsychotics and repeatedly relapsed into psychosis. He slashed his wrists and took an overdose in 1968. The next year, the police brought the patient to the hospital in restraints, and he was committed as a danger to others.

In both 1970 and 1971, he was committed after he threatened to rape his landlord's wife. He was then certified as "dangerous, mentally ill, hostile and combative" (3, p. 1067). He physically attacked several hospital employees. He was rehospitalized later in 1971 as violent and abusive. After the patient was charged with disorderly conduct and admitted in 1972, hospital psychiatrists noted that he was dangerous to himself and others, especially if he were to drive a car in his present condition. In 1973, he was admitted to Delaware State Hospital for the fifth time after intentionally ramming a police vehicle with his car. He was discharged and rehospitalized after he discontinued medication. Discharged again in 1973, he attempted suicide by setting fire to a tire in his apartment, hoping the fumes would kill him—his sixth Delaware State hospitalization. In 1974, he was hospitalized as homicidal and suicidal after driving his car off the road at a high speed. He rolled the car and gashed his left hand, sustaining permanent damage. After attempting to drown himself in 1975, he was again admitted.

The last hospitalization occurred after he locked himself in a hotel room. Again the police brought him in. He was committed, but then agreed to be a voluntary patient. Ten days later, he stopped taking his medication. The next day he requested discharge. Five days later, he was discharged. The psychiatrist, along with the treatment team, reviewed a digest and compilation of the patient's prior records and determined he was not committable. He was discharged with a 30-day supply of medication and given an appointment at the VA hospital.

He apparently never took his medication and never kept the appointment. He left the state, and five and one-half months later, while in a psychotic state, he caused a head-on automobile accident that resulted in the death of the plaintiff's husband.

The jury found the plaintiff's expert persuasive. He testified that the psychiatrist was grossly negligent in discharging the patient on very high doses of medication without a program for continued care and without an early outpatient appointment. The plaintiff's expert also testified that the psychiatrist failed to address the patient's inconsistent medication compliance and failed to consider alternatives such as referral to an outpatient facility, transfer to a VA hospital, or civil commitment. The jury found the defendant psychiatrist liable.

The Delaware Supreme Court affirmed the verdict. APA submitted an amicus brief, arguing that there were public policy reasons to overturn this verdict, namely that psychiatrists cannot predict dangerousness, and that cases like these will discourage psychiatrists from treating dangerous patients. The court found these arguments unconvincing.

In my opinion and in that of other public-sector psychiatrists, this case represents a system failure. There are patients who should not be in the community. On the facts, this man is clearly one of them. Given that, it is reasonable to compensate the plaintiff's decedent. Whether this psychiatrist should have been found grossly negligent on these facts can be debated. He paid the price for a longtime system failure in which he was one of many actors.

I suspect that many public-sector psychiatrists could have found themselves in Dr. Naidu's position. Working in a facility in which there is a premium on discharging patients because resources are limited, there is constant pressure to retain only those patients who are acutely psychotic or grossly disturbed. Courts have recognized those pressures in some cases, but in finding negligence, they focus on failure to make timely referrals to outpatient aftercare treatment. Had Dr. Naidu made a more timely referral, it might have protected him from this adverse verdict. In any case, psychiatrists who work in similar circumstances should strive always to make timely referrals for aftercare treatment.

Outpatient cases. *Schuster v. Altenberg* (15) is the *Tarasoff* case of first impression in Wisconsin. It is a troubling opinion for psychiatry. Currently, the Wisconsin Supreme Court has stated the legal duty and remanded the case for trial on the facts.

The published facts are sketchy. The allegedly manic-depressive patient caused an automobile accident in which she was killed and her daughter became paraplegic. Her widowed husband sued the doctor on behalf of his injured daughter, asking for substantial money for medical expenses and damages. He claimed the doctor was negligent in failing to warn the patient's family of her condition or its dangerous implications, in failing to warn of medication side effects, and in failing to commit the patient.

The court said negligent treatment or diagnosis can cause harm to a patient or a third party. Therefore, a third party can sue a physician for negligence.

The court then considered the question of liability for injuries resulting from medication side effects and decided the doctor could be liable if the doctor failed to properly warn the patient about the side effects. The court quoted several cases in which bus drivers on medication caused accidents, apparently as a result of medication side effects, and physicians were sued.

In Wisconsin, the court opined, a party is negligent if it was foreseeable that the party's act or omission to act could cause harm to someone. Therefore, under Wisconsin law, there is a duty to protect everyone, whether identifiable or not. Once the doctor or psychotherapist is found to be negligent, he or she is liable for any and all consequent harm caused by the negligent conduct:

> In the instant case, if it is ultimately proven that it would have been foreseeable to a psychiatrist, exercising due care, that by failing to warn a third person or by failing to take action to institute detention or commitment proceedings someone would be harmed, negligence will be established. (15, p. 240)

The court went on to consider public policy reasons against this opinion, rejecting all of them.

This opinion means that in Wisconsin there is now an affirmative duty to commit. This is different from the law in most jurisdictions that states that a physician may commit under certain conditions. Moreover, there is a duty to protect in Wisconsin that, if breached, can lead to a finding of negligence for any injury to anyone. The practical result is that liability will hang on testimony of competing experts.

This decision is quite inimical to the practice of psychiatry. Fortunately, no other recent opinion remotely resembles this one.

Discussion

The review of these and other cases suggests that courts are gradually increasing their understanding of the clinical issues. More and more courts are limiting duty to protect to cases in which the victim is clearly identifiable. Courts are explicitly rejecting the theory of *Lipari* that psychiatrists are liable to everyone for patient violence. The *Schuster* decision stands alone.

There is only one new published case in which a psychiatrist was found liable (3), and that is balanced by one old case in which a judgment on liability was set aside (5). In spite of the relatively few findings of liability, psychotherapists of all persuasions continue to be haunted by the fear of *Tarasoff*. This fear is consistent with findings in studies on risks associated with technological change: people tend to overestimate the risk of events that are dramatic and not under the individual's control, regardless of how frequently they occur (16). Large *Tarasoff* verdicts fit that description. They are rare, dramatic, and beyond the individual's control—exactly the kind of risk that people most overestimate.

In response to the perceived threat posed by *Tarasoff*, psychotherapists of all disciplines have pressed campaigns in many states to enact laws limiting liability (17). Such laws exist in at least a dozen states. All have in common that the duty to protect is limited to those cases in which a patient threatens an identifiable or reasonably identifiable victim. The therapist is excused from any liability if he or she carries out certain acts, such as warning the victim and/or the police, or hospitalizing the patient. Statutes vary, and readers should consult their local professional society to ascertain the law in their own jurisdiction.

The intent of these laws is to limit liability, and this has obvious advantages for the professions. However, there is a danger that therapists will adopt a cookbook approach to these problems based on following the letter of the law. This is unlikely to protect psychotherapists.

In general, courts are practical. The duty to protect calls on psychotherapists to exercise their professional judgment and then take whatever steps are reasonably necessary to prevent foreseeable harm. If professionals fail to exercise their judgment, imagining that they are excused from so doing by statute, they run serious risks. If a patient seriously injures someone, and the patient's therapist failed to exercise due care, the courts will find a way to hold the therapist liable, statutes notwithstanding.

The duty to protect exists to ensure that psychotherapists will deal responsibly with threats of violence. These are difficult cases, involving balancing of conflicting responsibilities and requiring thoughtful exercise of clinical judgment. The existence of statutes does not ease the clinical problems inherent in these cases.

In any case of threatened serious harm, the best defense against liability is the careful, unhurried exercise of sound clinical judgment. Too often therapists faced with a potentially violent patient jump from a consideration of the clinical problem to a defense posture designed to ward off the danger of suit. In the next chapter, Dr. Robert I. Simon discusses in some detail clinical strategies for assessing and dealing with the potentially violent patient.

Here it is important to note only two essential points. First, whenever possible—and this means in almost every case—the therapist should discuss his or her concerns with the patient. The therapist should approach threatened violence as a clinical task requiring consideration by the therapist and the patient working together. Preventing violence is in the patient's interest as well as in the interest of the potential victim and the therapist.

Second, it is essential when confronted with potential violence that the therapist carefully document the encounter. Too often therapists do good work but fail to make a careful record of their observations. In cases of this kind, therapists should record not only their observations but their conclusions, their proposed course of action, and the rationale for the course they chose and for the alternatives they rejected. The therapist with a well-developed sense of self-preservation should always make time to write this kind of careful note whenever the case involves potential violence to the patient or anyone else.

References

1. Jablonski v U.S., 712 F2d 391 (9th Cir 1983)
2. Peck v The Counseling Service of Addison County, 499 A2d 422 (Vt 1985)
3. Naidu v Laird, 539 A2d 1064 (Del Sup Ct 1988)
4. Davis v Lhim, 335 NW2d 481, 124 (Mich App 291 1983)
5. Canon v Thumudo, 422 NW2d 688 (Mich 1988)
6. Novak v Rathnam, 505 NE2d 773 (Ill App 1987)
7. Phillips v Roy, 94 So2d 1342 (La Ct App 1986)
8. Cooke v Berlin, 735 P2d 830 (Ariz Ct App 1987)
9. Lipari v Sears, 497 FSupp 185 (D Neb 1980)
10. Petersen v Washington, 671 P2d 230, 100 (Wash 421 1983)
11. Bardoni v Kim, 390 NW2d 218 (Mich App 1986)
12. Paul v Plymouth General Hospital, 408 NW2d 492 (Mich Ct App 1987)
13. Hinkelman v Borgess Medical Center, 403 NW2d 547 (Mich App 1987)

14. Pangborn v Saad, 326 SE2d 365 (NC App 1985)
15. Schuster v Altenberg, 424 NW2d 159, 87-0115 (Wisc Sup Ct 1988)
16. Slovic P, Fischhoff B, Lichtenstein S: Behavioral decision theory perspectives on risk and safety. Acta Psychologica 56:183–203, 1984
17. Appelbaum PS, Zonana H, Bonnie R, et al: Statutory approaches to limiting psychiatrists' liability for their patients' violent acts. Am J Psychiatry 146:821–828, 1989

CHAPTER THREE

The Duty to Protect
in Private Practice

Robert I. Simon, M.D.

Inevitably, psychiatrists in private practice must treat violent mentally ill patients in their offices. The only way to avoid these patients is to not take *any* patients. Beck (1) observed that psychiatrists in private practice often lack experience in treating violent patients. Furthermore, *Tarasoff* cases in private practice more often end in violence or ruptured therapeutic relationships than in other settings. Beck concluded that the threat of violence is a greater problem for the psychiatrist practicing in the office than previously suspected. Nothing unnerves psychiatrists and disrupts their free-floating attention more than patients who make threats of violence toward others.

Initially, individuals who present themselves for treatment may appear to be free of violent tendencies. But it is the rare patient who does not have to struggle, to some degree or another, with violent thoughts and feelings directed toward self or others. The clinician must be able to systematically assess a patient's risk of violence to others. In this chapter, I will present two hypothetical clinical case examples that illustrate a method for violence assessment.

Predicting Violent Behavior

Dangerousness, as used here, refers to the potential for violence. When the proper conditions or circumstances arise, potential violence can become actual violence. One might think of all individuals as dangerous under some circumstances. A parent whose child is recklessly endangered may react violently. Violence may be an appropriate self-protective reaction in certain situations.

Studies demonstrate that the dangerousness of psychiatric patients is equivalent to that of persons in the general population (2). For psychiatric clinicians, dangerousness is a function of the dynamic interaction between a specific individual and a given situation during a limited period of time. Second-generation research on violence is clinically possible in some instances. Stone (3) stated that psychiatrists do have some expertise in determining from the mental status evaluation whether a patient manifests violent tendencies. However, predictions of dangerousness that extend beyond the current state of the patient have not been validated.

Predictive accuracy also may be improved for defined homogeneous populations having high base rates for violence. For example, a closed psychiatric unit containing very disturbed patients may have violence base rates of 25–35%. Actuarial data containing known base rates for specific groups are an important assessment variable.

The best protection against allegations of negligence when making predictions of dangerousness is to evaluate violence according to methods and procedures that take into account known variables associated with violence (Table 1). Because the psychiatrist is likely to be wrong two out of three times, humility dictates careful documentation of how the assessment of violence was conducted.

Violence Variables

Personal, socioeconomic, situational, and clinical variables are associated with violence. Monahan (4) has shown the association of violence with being male, black, and ages 15–20 years; with having employment and residential instability; and with a history of alcohol or drug abuse and previous violence. Situational factors associated with violence include an unstable family, a violent environment, a violent peer group, and availability of weapons and victims.

Clinical variables associated with violence include a history of violence, soft neurological signs, low intelligence, impulsivity (e.g., previous violence toward self or others, reckless driving, unrestrained spending), paranoid ideation, command hallucinations, psychosis, and the stated desire to hurt or kill another. The ther-

Table 1. Assessment of violence: risk variables for Case Example 1

Risk variables	Facilitating violence	Inhibiting violence
Motive	H	
Therapeutic alliance (ongoing patient)	H	
Other relationships	H	
Psychiatric diagnosis (Axis I and II)	H	
Situational status	0	0
Employment status		M
Actuarial data (age, sex, race, socioeconomic group, marital status, violence base rates)	L	
Availability of lethal means	H	
Available victim	H	
Syntonic or dystonic violence	H	
Specific plan	H	
Specific person threatened	H	
Past violent acts[a]	H	
Childhood abuse (or witnessing spouse abuse)	M	
Alcohol abuse	0	0
Drug abuse	0	0
Mental competence	M	
History of impulsive behavior	M	
Central nervous system disorder		H
Low intelligence		M

Note. Use rating system: L = low factor; M = moderate factor; H = high factor; 0 = nonfactor. Clinically judge low, medium, or high potential for violence within 24–48 hours based on assessment of violence.
[a]When a specific person is threatened and past violence has occurred, a high risk potential for violence rating is achieved.

apeutic alliance can be a very effective deterrent to violence. However, with new patients or patients seen in emergencies, sufficient time may not have elapsed for an alliance to form. Rarely does the therapist have an alliance with the victim.

A constellation of factors have been identified in young persons that should alert mental health professionals to a high potential for future violence. These include serious violence as a juvenile, psychotic symptoms, major neurological impairment and head injury, abuse as a child, witnessing one family member abuse another,

Table 2. Potential for violence and suggested psychiatric intervention

Potential for violence	Psychiatric interventions
High	Immediate hospitalization if mentally ill and likely to benefit from hospitalization
Medium	Hospitalization
	Frequent outpatient visits, consider warning and calling the police
	Reevaluate patient and treatment plan frequently
	Remain available to the patient
Low	Continue with current treatment plan

Note. Tables 1 and 2 represent only one method of violence risk assessment and intervention. The purpose of these tables is heuristic, encouraging a systematic approach to risk assessment. However, the therapist's clinical judgment concerning the patient remains paramount. Given the fact that violence risk factors will be assigned different weights according to the clinical presentation of the patient, these tables cannot be followed rigidly.

psychiatric hospitalization, or psychotic relatives. On the other hand, presence of obsessive-compulsive defenses may help increase internal controls.

Motive is an extremely important clinical variable in the assessment of violence (5). When patients respond affirmatively to questions about whether they would like to hurt someone, the therapist must ask "who, when, where, why, and how long?" Information gleaned from these inquiries is critical to the evaluation of the following questions: How imminent is the threat of violence? Who is the object of potential violence? What can be done to treat the patient and protect potential victims?

Careful assessment and documentation of pertinent clinical variables may prevent allegations of negligent assessment. Even if the therapist is tragically wrong in the prediction of violence, a mistake is not malpractice if a reasonable standard of care was utilized in predicting violence. Tables 1 and 2 demonstrate one method of assessment and intervention.

Tarasoff and Psychiatric Practice

The vast majority of courts have held that in outpatient cases, the therapist's control over the patient is not sufficient to establish a duty to protect unless there is a foreseeable victim. The danger must be substantial, involving serious bodily harm or death. If no threats or violent acts are uncovered after careful documented clinical evaluation, liability is unlikely should violence occur. By contrast, in inpatient release cases, several courts have held that there is a duty to control a patient with or without a foreseeable victim when there is reasonable evidence that the patient may be dangerous.

Beck (5) points out that after a clinical assessment reveals that the patient is potentially violent, three options are open: 1) deal with the violence in the therapy; 2) discuss the problem with a third person, such as the victim and/or the police; or 3) voluntarily or involuntarily hospitalize the patient. Like weather forecasts, short-term assessments of potential for violence are more accurate than long-term forecasts because the parameters that influence future occurrences can be specified with greater precision. For predictions made at a greater distance, the clinician loses the ability to specify both psychological and environmental determinants of behavior and thus the ability to predict with precision the likelihood of particular outcomes. Accordingly, potentially violent patients should be seen face to face frequently and their risks for violence reassessed each time. Assessment is not an academic exercise. Its sole purpose is to guide patient management. Appelbaum (6) aptly stated: "Clinicians have learned to live with *Tarasoff*, recognizing that good common sense, sound clinical practice, careful documentation, and a genuine concern for their patients are almost always sufficient to fulfill their legal obligations" (p. 106).

Risk-Benefit Assessment

For any treatment intervention with a potentially violent patient, the clinician should conduct and immediately record a risk-benefit assessment. A documented risk-benefit analysis that considers clinically relevant interventions with dangerous patients will be useful in demonstrating that reasonable care was taken with the patient, even if there is a violent outcome. Categorical statements that the patient is no longer dangerous are less legally defensible than notes that take into account the assessment of the relevant risk variables in judging the *potential* for violence balanced against the benefits of a particular treatment intervention. Verbatim notes provide the best evidence to support clinical conclusions. A note should conclude with a statement about the likelihood of violence, a proposed course of action, and the reasoning behind the interventions chosen and those considered and rejected, citing the clinical data relied on.

Consultation with a colleague may be reassuring to both the patient and the therapist. The consultant should document the consultation. An informal consultation can take place over the telephone, if necessary; although not ideal, it is better than no consultation at all. The psychiatrist should summarize the consultant's opinion in the patient's record. If legal questions arise later, consultation may help establish that a reasonable standard of care was provided to the patient. Psychiatric residents should consider increasing the frequency of their supervision when a dangerous patient is undergoing a crisis. If time allows, decisions regarding management of the dangerous patient should be endorsed with the supervisor's signature.

Assessing the Potential for Violence

Assessing violence according to a reasonable standard of care can be done anywhere. Based on the assessment of risk variables, a probability determination of low, medium, or high potential for violence can be made according to a tabulation of clinical factors that increase or decrease the risk of violence. These probability determinations, like predictions of the weather, are only relevant to the immediate future—hours or days—not weeks or months. Therefore, they should be updated frequently (see Tables 1 and 2). The potential for violence is a clinical judgment call for which no clear standards exist. Certainly, the accurate prediction of a specific violent act is not currently possible.

The assessment of dangerousness contains two separate parts: gathering information and evaluating the probability of a future violent act. Appelbaum (6) suggests that two questions be routinely asked: "Have you ever seriously injured another person?" and "Do you ever think about harming someone else?" These two questions often yield surprising information not obtained from the general psychiatric history. The most common mistake that clinicians make is insufficient gathering of information on which a later determination of dangerousness is based. When confronted with the violent patient, the clinician should attempt to deepen the evaluation to include closer scrutiny of defenses, conflicts, and other psychodynamic issues. Although a standard of care does not exist for predicting dangerousness, clear standards do exist for gathering sufficient information for satisfying a reasonable standard of care. Since prediction is so problematic, careful documentation from visit to visit of the clinical reasoning behind the decision concerning dangerousness is essential when violence is threatened.

Selecting a Course of Action

Selecting a course of action depends on the clinical needs of the violent patient and the ingenuity of the therapist. Although too many options to list here, they can include incorporating the potential victim into the therapy, utilizing voluntary and involuntary hospitalization, and seeking social service interventions to improve the environmental situation. Follow-up must be adequate but is limited by the patient's cooperation. If the patient stops taking medication or drops out of treatment, these issues should be addressed aggressively. The psychiatrist should call or write the patient who precipitously terminates therapy. In ongoing therapy, interventions should be reevaluated. If they have failed to alter the patient's tendency toward violence, new interventions should be tried. If the patient is transferred to another facility, the assessment of dangerousness must be communicated. Reassessment for dangerousness must be made before discharge.

After a petition for civil commitment, responsibility passes to the judicial system. If the court deems the patient not committable and the patient ultimately harms someone, no liability should attach to the clinician. Nevertheless, the therapist should go on record as opposing discharge of a violent mentally ill patient.

Case Example 1

A 45-year-old nuclear physicist specializing in nuclear weapons development had been in individual psychotherapy for 3 months.

He developed a reactive depression after the breakup of a love affair.

During the course of treatment, the psychiatrist learned that the patient's mother died when he was 3 years old. His father was an alcoholic and physically abused the patient. The patient remembers that, as a child, he felt very rejected, hurt, and frightened by his feelings of helplessness and storms of rage. Although his father remarried when the patient was 5, his stepmother was cold and distant. He received much of his early sense of worth through academic achievement and the praise of teachers. He was an honor student in college and graduate school, winning many academic awards. However, in his personal relationships, he remained aloof and was known as a loner.

After receiving his doctorate, the patient stayed with the physics department of his university until an argument with the chairman of the department caused him to leave. He became depressed at that time, seeking the help of a psychotherapist. The psychiatrist knew of this previous treatment but did not obtain the records from the former therapist. The treatment records would have revealed that the patient had attempted to choke the department chairman during their argument, requiring physical restraint by others.

The patient's initial depression abated when he was asked to take an important research position with a prestigious institution that received grants for the development of nuclear weapons. Although uncertain about whether to work with weapons development, he eventually decided to take the position. The patient created a breakthrough with his discovery and development of very small nuclear weapons. These weapons were extremely valuable for use in military war games and against selected targets where highly circumscribed lethality was required.

While working on this project, the patient became enamored of his secretary. She was 20 years younger than the patient and had worked for him about a year before their personal relationship developed. For the first time in his life, the patient felt happy and close to another human being. His hobby was collecting guns, and the couple spent many hours together firing his treasured weapons. However, her family was against her dating the patient because they considered him odd. Six months after the relationship began, it dissolved when she resigned her position as his secretary and refused to see him. She had become alarmed by his jealous rages and his desires for bondage and other sadistic practices in their sexual relationship. The patient was devastated and slipped back into depression.

The psychiatrist diagnosed reactive depression. There were no vegetative signs. Three-times-a-week psychotherapy was begun. After 2 months of therapy, the patient decided to cut back to once-a-week therapy. He received a major promotion that temporarily ameliorated his depression. The psychiatrist was concerned that the patient had not dealt with his feelings of anger and loss.

The psychiatrist also questioned the possible transference implications of the patient's decision to cut back appointments. The psychiatrist, a woman, recalled that the patient's mother died when he was 3 years old and that his stepmother was a cold and distant figure. Did the patient fear his hostile feelings toward women? Was he afraid of getting too close and exposing vulnerable, tender feelings? The psychiatrist felt that her patient could not tolerate transference interpretations at this point.

Three weeks after his decision to cut back therapy, the patient rapidly slipped into a profound depression and developed the delusion that death by cancer was imminent. The psychiatrist was alarmed by the patient's ideas that his former girlfriend, her parents, and his former department head at the university were gloating over his imminent demise. He had never been able to settle his guilt over developing nuclear weapons and now felt that his upcoming death was punishment. He spent much time going over his gun collection, ruminating about whether death by his own hand was preferable to a frightening death by cancer. He told the psychiatrist that just before that appointment, the idea struck him that perhaps he should die by the very weapons he had engineered and "take some of the other worthless people with me." Also during that past week, the patient had made threatening calls to his former girlfriend, her parents, and his former department chairman, identifying himself. The psychiatrist proposed a return to three-times-a-week psychotherapy and the starting of antidepressant medication. He refused both suggestions, saying, "I am going to die soon anyway." The patient did not want drugs to confuse his thinking or interfere with his "final plans." The psychiatrist's recommendation of psychiatric hospitalization was viewed by the patient as a plot by his enemies to "foil me."

The psychiatrist knew that the patient had access to small nuclear weapons with a force of approximately 1,000 pounds of TNT, enough destructive power to kill anyone within 500 feet of ground zero. Radiation and heat were lethal up to 1,000 feet. The weapon was considered "clean" but could still cause radiation sickness to significant numbers of people. Also, for the first time, the patient was considering carrying a .380-caliber Beretta pistol. He was not eating well and had lost 10 pounds in the past 2 weeks. Much of his nights was spent "pacing and plotting." The psychiatrist performed an assessment of this patient's risk for violence. Table 1 shows the variables assessed and their values for this patient. The rating for potential violence is high.

The psychiatrist was reasonably familiar with the Tarasoff case and some of its progeny. She knew that in her jurisdiction, no Tarasoff-type case had been decided. Furthermore, a strict confidentiality statute, with few exceptions, prohibited disclosure of information without the patient's consent. The psychiatrist was concerned that because of the patient's delusional depression, he might attempt to kill the three individuals he had threatened or perpetrate mass murder through a nuclear disaster. The psychiatrist decided to test the therapeutic alliance at this critical point by urging the patient to accept voluntary hospitalization. He refused. The psychiatrist straightforwardly informed the patient that she could not allow him to remain untreated and dangerous to himself and others. She stated that she would file for an involuntary hospitalization if he refused voluntary hospitalization. He shouted "traitor" and rushed out of the office.

The psychiatrist now considered her options (see Table 2). She reasoned that because no duty to protect law existed in her state and because the three individuals threatened were fully aware of the threats made against them by the patient, no need existed to warn them. Although a strict confidentiality statute existed, she decided that the danger to others was so great that ethically, morally, and professionally she must inform the police. In addition, the psychiatrist signed medical certification papers for involuntary hospitalization of the patient, which permitted the police to apprehend *the patient at home and take him to a designated psychiatric hospital. The psychiatrist canceled her remaining appointments, knowing she could not concentrate on listening to her patients and wanting to devote full time to following through on this case.*

Demonstration of Violence Assessment Techniques

Applying the assessment of violence risk variables in Table 1 to the case example, the following analysis can be made. The patient's motive in wanting to inflict violence is clear—a projected sense of guilt and worthlessness as well as a desire for revenge (rating *motive*: high—facilitating violence). The therapeutic alliance between the patient and the psychiatrist has become a negative force, i.e., the patient feels betrayed and persecuted by the psychiatrist (rating *therapeutic alliance*: high—facilitating violence). Apart from his former girlfriend and the psychiatrist, the patient has not had any other sustaining relationships. These relationships are not now available to him. He perceives the psychiatrist as his enemy (rating *other relationships*: high—facilitating violence). A major depression with psychotic features appears to be the most likely Axis I diagnosis (DSM-III-R). The Axis II diagnosis is personality disorder not otherwise specified with mixed borderline and schizoid features (rating *psychiatric diagnosis*: high—facilitating violence). The external situation precipitating the depression appears to be the breakup with his girlfriend, which occurred approximately 3 months before this evaluation. Negative transference developments appear to be the most important subsequent change in the patient's status but should be subsumed under the rating for the therapeutic alliance. Situational status refers to immediate external environmental factors that could precipitate violence, such as a violent environment or a threat of violence by another. This does not appear to be a factor (rating *situational status*: 0—nonfactor).

The patient's employment status has been stable throughout his life. He has been recognized for his achievements and promoted to positions of responsibility. Although the patient has remained ambivalent about his work with armaments, particularly nuclear weapons, his employment status must be considered a stabilizing factor (rating *employment status*: moderate—inhibiting violence).

Actuarial data including age, sex, race, socioeconomic group, marital status, and violence base rates are not particularly helpful in evaluating this patient. No violence base rate exists for his socioeconomic or occupational group. At 45 years of age, race becomes an even more controversial issue than for ages 15–20. Male gender may be the only actuarial factor of some relevance for predicting violence in this case (rating *actuarial data*: low—facilitating violence).

The patient is a gun enthusiast with access to his gun collection. At the time of the evaluation, the patient is considering carrying a .380-caliber Beretta pistol (rating *availability of lethal means*: high—facilitating violence). All of the threatened victims are available because their whereabouts are known to the patient (rating *available victim*: high—facilitating violence). Violence can usually be specified as syntonic or dystonic from the patient's perspective. The patient does not perceive his violent impulses and threats toward others as alien. On the contrary, violence toward others is appealing to the patient (rating *syntonic or dystonic violence*: high—facilitating violence). The patient has enunciated a plan using micronuclear weapons to kill others. He has access to such weapons. The patient does not want to take drugs that could confuse his thinking and interfere with his violent plans (rating *specific plan*: high—facilitating violence). The patient threatens three individuals directly with telephone calls, identifying himself. Whenever a specific person is threatened and has a history of past violent acts, a high risk potential for violence is automatically achieved.

The patient was physically abused as a child, although the full extent of the abuse is unknown at the time of psychiatric evaluation (rating *childhood abuse*: moderate—facilitating violence). Alcohol and drug abuse are not part of the clinical picture (rating *alcohol and drug abuse*: 0—nonfactors). In this case, the evaluation of mental competence is tricky. From a narrow legal, cognitive perspective, the patient would probably be considered competent. However, due to the presence of a severe delusional depression, the patient is affectively incompetent clinically; that is, the depression interferes significantly with the patient's reality testing (rating *mental competence*: moderate—facilitating violence). Impulsive behavior occurred once before when the patient attempted to choke his department chairman. With borderline personality features as part of the Axis II diagnosis, potential for impulsive behavior exists (rating *history of impulsive behavior*: moderate—facilitating violence). The patient has no diagnosis of a central nervous system (CNS) disorder. High rather than low intelligence characterizes the patient. Nevertheless, high intelligence can be put in the service of violence when under the sway of an affective disorder. However, on balance, the patient's intelligence, which he has lived by most of his life, must be considered a mitigating factor (rating *CNS disorder*: high—inhibiting violence; rating *low intelligence*: moderate—inhibiting violence).

A review of Table 1 leads to an unequivocal assessment of high violence potential for the patient. The most appropriate psychiatric intervention is clearly immediate hospitalization. It must be stressed that hospitalization of violent individuals should only occur when they have a diagnosable mental illness and appear likely to benefit from psychiatric hospitalization. Psychiatrists are not the police officers of society and should not attempt to hospitalize nonmentally ill violent persons who are unlikely to benefit from available treatments.

Conclusion of Case Example 1

The designated psychiatric hospital for involuntary hospitalizations received the patient from the police. By law, the hospital had 72 hours to evaluate the patient and make a dispositional recommendation. The patient agreed to a transfer to another hospital where he would be a voluntary patient under the care of his former psychiatrist. Within a few days, the therapeutic alliance with the former psychiatrist was restored. After 6 weeks of hospitalization on 200 mg of imipramine per day, the patient had a complete remission of his delusional depression. At discharge, the patient was not experiencing any violent thoughts or feelings. The patient continued outpatient treatment twice weekly for a year with excellent results.

Summary

The psychiatrist's management of the patient could have been enhanced by obtaining the prior psychiatric record. Thus, with the information about prior violence, the psychiatrist might have better anticipated the patient's threats of violence. Also, she would have had more time to consult with an attorney or forensic colleague. Should a psychiatrist warn potential victims even when they are aware of the threat? Does a warning from a psychiatrist have a greater impact, and thus, is it more likely to be heeded? Given the psychiatrist's knowledge of the patient's background of physical abuse and his hobby of collecting guns and developing weapons, should the psychiatrist have explored therapeutically the possible connections between the meaning of weapons to the patient's feelings of hurt, fear, helplessness, and anger? If the transference was turning negative, should the psychiatrist have given priority to managing the negative transference therapeutically, perhaps offering an interpretation at a level the patient could accept?

The fact that no *Tarasoff*-type duty to warn exists in the psychiatrist's state should not be a determinative factor. The psychiatrist correctly reasoned that her ethical, moral, and professional duty dictated that she try to protect both her patient and other potential victims by calling the police. She used similar reasoning in breaching the confidentiality statute. She did not merely call the police and then go about her business as usual. She recognized that she was upset and that she could not ignore the worries and fears raised by this case. She decided to cancel the rest of her patients so that she would be available as needed.

Follow-up to see that recommended interventions have been implemented is very important. Therapists must be able to tolerate disruptions of their schedule, loss of time and money, and their own feelings of anger and frustration occasioned by the clinical and legal difficulties surrounding the management of violent, threatening patients.

With an ever-increasing number of states adopting *Tarasoff* in their court rulings, including some states by statutory provision (7), therapists cannot assume legal invulnerability from victim suits in states that have not yet adopted *Tarasoff* principles into law. Given this ambiguity, the best policy in the treatment of potentially violent patients is to practice with extreme care, to be aware of statutory or case law in the state where one practices, or if no state law exists, to be aware of national trends in the law. There is no guarantee, however, that what has legally transpired in other states will be recapitulated in similar form in one's own state.

Case Example 2

For the past 6 months, a 43-year-old woman with a (DSM-III-R) Axis I diagnosis of dysthymic disorder and an Axis II diagnosis of dependent personality disorder has been seen in twice-per-week psychotherapy. The patient is a very successful accountant. No medications have been prescribed. A central theme in the treatment has been the suppression and denial of her rage. The psychiatrist has a good working alliance with the patient.

The patient has been married for 6 years and has a 3-year-old daughter. During the past year and a half, her alcoholic corporate executive husband has become increasingly physically abusive. On one occasion, he knocked two of his wife's teeth loose and on another struck her on the head with a baseball bat, causing a laceration and a mild concussion. The patient confided this history of abuse to a number of her close friends who have been of considerable support to her. While the patient has long suffered because of marked dependency needs and a history of physical abuse as a child, she has increasingly harbored fantasies of revenge toward her husband. After the last episode of physical abuse 2 weeks ago when the husband injured her shoulder by twisting her arm, she threatened to kill him. She spoke with a favorite uncle, who is a sportsman, about purchasing one of his guns. The husband refused all requests by the psychiatrist to come for an interview either individually or with his wife. When the husband inadvertently learned about his wife's request to purchase a gun, he threatened to strangle her.

The patient now fears for her own life. Though never violent in the past, she is determined to protect herself if her husband abuses her again. She sends her daughter to stay temporarily with an aunt. The patient is increasingly beset by unbidden murderous impulses toward her husband and frightening nightmares involving his dismemberment. There is no evidence of psychosis. She reluctantly purchases a gun from her uncle.

The psychiatrist determines that the patient requires immediate psychiatric intervention, but the patient refuses psychiatric hospitalization. The psychiatrist considers the following options: warn the husband, call the police, seek immediate medical certification for involuntary civil commitment, see the patient more frequently, and/or begin pharmacotherapy. A duty to protect statute has been *recently enacted in this state, limiting the liability of psychotherapists whose patients harm others and requiring the psychotherapist to warn an identifiable victim and to notify the police of the danger.*

Assessment of Violence

Applying the violence risk variables contained in Table 1 to the patient in Case Example 2, a high rating for violence toward her husband is achieved despite the presence of significant inhibiting factors. To become familiar with this method of violence risk assessment, readers may wish to make their own assessments of the patients presented in the case examples.

Referring to Table 2, the psychiatric intervention most frequently associated with a high rating for violence is immediate hospitalization. But, as can be seen from later discussion, the psychiatrist chose an alternative tailored to the needs of this patient.

Warning Endangered Third Parties

Issuing a warning as a legal formalism is not an acceptable approach to managing the violent patient. Though at least 13 states have defined the *Tarasoff* duty by statute and narrowed the potential liability, the psychiatrist who does not exercise reasonable professional judgment in managing the violent patient may still be vulnerable to a suit. Therapists must be reasonably certain that the threat of harm to others is imminent. Moreover, reasonable efforts to control the patient must be made before issuing a warning to the intended victim. If a warning is issued, reasonable follow-up should be attempted.

Generally, when the therapist decides to warn potential victims, a telephone call is appropriate so that the potential victim can ask questions. Telephoning in the patient's presence helps temper exaggerated remarks by the therapist, who may be overreacting to the threat of violence. Additionally, the patient's presence tends to head off psychotic or paranoid ideas that the psychiatrist is acting duplicitously. The warning should be clear, as some courts have criticized the clarity of the warning.

How—not whether—the warning is given is crucial. When the clinician discusses the warning with the patient before giving it, the clinical result is usually positive. Not discussing the warning with the patient almost always turns out badly for the therapeutic alliance and the therapy. Potential victims should be warned in a clinically supportive manner. If the victim feels evasive action can be taken and the therapist is acting in a responsible, concerned manner, the warning is likely to be received positively.

The psychology of victim-victimizer husband-wife or partner relationships may dictate attempting to move the victim toward a sheltered environment rather than warning the abuser that the abused partner is considering retaliatory violence. To do otherwise might seriously endanger the patient or precipitate mutual violence. This is precisely the point of the case example. Warning the patient's abuser could precipitate more violence toward the patient.

Conclusion of Case Example 2

After pondering the fact that his patient has purchased a gun to implement her murderous feelings, the psychiatrist first decides to obtain a forensic consultation. In a telephone consultation, the forensic psychiatrist suggests first that the patient be temporarily moved to a sheltered environment before warning the husband and calling the police. The consultant recommends a social worker familiar with sheltered environments for abused women.

The social worker then arranges admission of the patient to a sheltered home, and the patient is relieved. The psychiatrist sees his patient more frequently during this crisis, also prescribing some antianxiety medication. Together, the psychiatrist and the patient determine a plan of action. With the psychiatrist also on the telephone, the patient calls her husband and informs him that she purchased a gun and that she will notify the police of his abuse. The psychiatrist identifies himself on the telephone to the husband, confirming the patient's feelings of anger and wishes for revenge. At the conclusion of this conversation, the psychiatrist and the patient call the police. She informs the police that she has been a longstanding victim of physical abuse by her husband and that she has purchased a gun to protect herself. The psychiatrist also informs the police that the situation is very volatile and that the patient has been admitted to a sheltered home. The patient agrees to turn over her gun to the police. The crisis is temporarily defused.

Summary

Case Example 2 illustrates two essential points. First, warning is only one of the many measures the clinician can utilize in protecting endangered third parties from violent patients. However, reflexive warning, without regard for the clinical situation of the patient, ends badly for everyone. Second, the psychiatrist did not abrogate his clinical judgment in order to accommodate a statute. Instead, statutory requirements were met within the context of clinical interventions that were appropriate for the needs of the patient.

Conclusion

The psychiatrist in private practice will inevitably encounter patients who pose the threat of violence toward others. A systematic method of violence assessment will assist the psychiatrist to appropriately manage these difficult patients. Psychiatrists in private practice may not be able to obtain a consultation as quickly as may be necessary. In lieu of a consultation, applying a systematic approach to the assessment of the risk of violence also can ensure that the standard of care for the assessment of violence has been met.

References

1. Beck JC: Violent patients and the *Tarasoff* duty in private practice. Journal of Psychiatry and Law 23:361–376, 1985
2. Kamenar PD: Psychiatrists' duty to warn of a dangerous patient: survey of the law. Behavioral Sciences and the Law 2:259–272, 1984
3. Stone AA: Law, Psychiatry, and Morality. Washington, DC, American Psychiatric Press, 1984
4. Monahan J: The clinical prediction of violent behavior (DHHS Publ No ADM-81-921). Rockville, MD, National Institute of Mental Health, 1981
5. Beck JC: The potentially violent patient: legal duties, clinical practice, and risk management. Psychiatric Annals 17:695–699, 1987
6. Appelbaum PS: Implications of *Tarasoff* for clinical practice, in The

Potentially Violent Patient and the *Tarasoff* Decision in Psychiatric Practice. Edited by Beck JC. Washington, DC, American Psychiatric Press, 1985, pp 93–108
7. Appelbaum PS, Zonana H, Bonnie R, et al: Statutory approaches to limiting psychiatrists' liability for their patients' violent acts. Am J Psychiatry 146:821–828, 1989

CHAPTER FOUR

The Duty to Protect in Emergency Psychiatry

Kimberly A. White, M.D.
James C. Beck, M.D., Ph.D.

P sychiatric emergency services are an integral part of the community mental health system. These services support outpatient clinics and office practitioners in their work with the mentally ill. They are in a unique position to see patients at their most acute or evolved stages of decompensation. Their staffs are trained and their space is designed to handle these difficult patients. The question of how to assess and treat patients who are dangerous arises daily for emergency room psychiatrists. For that reason, the *Tarasoff* decision has great relevance to this crisis work (1,2).

Emergency psychiatry is both similar to and different from psychiatric work in other clinical settings. To begin with the similarities, the emergency room setting shares with other psychiatric settings the long-established understanding of confidentiality between physician and patient (3). Emergency room psychiatrists have the same *Tarasoff* responsibility as other clinicians to protect potential victims from dangerous patients (4–6). Emergency room psychiatrists are equally vulnerable to suit if they wrongfully violate confidentiality or inadequately attend to protecting potential victims of their patients.

There has been controversy about the effect of *Tarasoff* on the therapeutic relationship. Several authors have asserted that the *Tarasoff* guidelines can be used to strengthen the therapeutic relationship, or at least to be a workable part of the therapy (7–9). Some authors stress that many conscientious therapists observed an ethical duty to protect even before *Tarasoff* (10,11). Other authors continue to express anxiety about integrating this responsibility with the confidentiality otherwise assumed in a therapeutic relationship. The debate is relevant to patient care issues in the psychiatric emergency room as well as in psychiatric practice generally.

Emergency room psychiatry differs from psychiatry in other settings. These differences contribute to an emergency service's conservative approach to the duty to protect. Special considerations in the emergency room include 1) the limitation of a one-time assessment in gathering all relevant data for each patient; 2) the difficulty in evaluating patients who present in the midst of a severe, floridly symptomatic episode rather than in the early stages before an episode becomes an emergency, or in an acutely dangerous condition; and 3) the lack of an ongoing alliance between the patient and emergency room staff. In fact, many emergency service patients have no prior relationship with any treating professional. These patients are often not motivated to follow treatment recommendations, and staff are often reluctant to refer them to less restrictive outpatient alternative treatment settings.

Additional sources of difficulty in the emergency room are the need for transfer of responsibility and care for most patients in implementing disposition and treatment plans and the emergence of a new group of dangerous, character-disordered and/or substance-abusing patients who fall on the line between traditional mental health services and the judicial system (12).

To offset the difficulties inherent in this work, emergency psychiatrists should freely use consultants, such as forensic experts, lawyers, and hospital administrators, for second opinions on difficult cases. Emergency room psychiatrists should always review whatever medical records are readily available. In at least one unpublished malpractice suit that followed a patient's suicide, the emergency physician's failure to review the patient's past record from the same hospital was alleged to be negligent.

Psychiatrists who work in these settings should be familiar with predictors of violence and expert in crisis assessment and management. Emergency clinicians must make the best assessment possible based on all the available information obtained in a discrete period of time.

There is one published case of emergency psychiatry in which the psychiatrist was found to be negligent (*Jablonski v. U.S.*) (4, 13–

15). This decision focused on the psychiatrist's not adequately gathering information—the psychiatrist did not review medical records documenting the patient's previous history of serious violence; not heeding police warnings of the patient's potential violence; and, finally, not adequately protecting the victim (who was murdered), although the psychiatrist warned her to stay away.

The *Jablonski* case emphasizes the responsibility of an emergency service to gather all available information and to take reasonable action to protect potential victims.

Case Example 1

When patients present to the emergency room, their condition is often an acute exacerbation of their underlying difficulties. Sometimes this is recognized by others, e.g., family, police, or therapist, and at other times it is the patient himself or herself who becomes concerned. Situations that concern an outpatient therapist may blossom into more acute, serious problems that come to emergency service staff attention before the therapist can reassess them. In other cases, a patient or situation becomes too dangerous for an outpatient therapist to manage alone.

The following case example demonstrates that *Tarasoff* guidelines can be used in a therapeutic clinical manner in crisis settings, even where there is no ongoing relationship between the emergency room or any other service provider and the patient.

T.N. is a 29-year-old employed, married man who referred himself to the psychiatric emergency room after a difficult day in probate court. He and his father were disputing an inheritance. In the emergency room, he complained of depression and "stress," and he feared he would lose control with his wife if he went home. He had been psychiatrically hospitalized for 3 days the previous week for similar complaints, but had left against medical advice. He was not in outpatient therapy.

He stated that he had not previously harmed his wife but that he was becoming increasingly angry at her frequent absences from their home at night, and her lack of attention to him and his current difficulties. He did not think there was any alternative but psychiatric hospitalization. He denied alcohol or drug abuse. He was diagnosed as adjustment disorder with mixed emotional features and threatened disturbance of conduct.

Because of his increasing agitation during his emergency room visit, staff physically restrained him and medicated him twice with a short-acting benzodiazepine. After reviewing his previous hospitalization with the inpatient team and discussing the proposed disposition with the patient, the emergency psychiatrist arranged commitment to the state hospital. She also discussed with the patient her wish to tell his wife of his concerns about his own potential violence and his hospitalization. Although he was initially reluctant, he gave permission for the psychiatrist to call his wife. The emergency psychiatrist told the patient's wife of his fears of losing control and harming her, and of plans to hospitalize him. After the psychiatrist spoke with his wife, the patient himself phoned her and tried to explain further his anger and fears of harming her. The psychiatrist documented her own concerns for his potential violence on his admission paperwork, and she spoke about them to the hospital doctor on call.

The psychiatrist hoped the discussion between the patient and his wife would speed up the clinical work that would follow in the hospital. If the patient had refused to contact his wife, the psychiatrist would not have felt obliged to do so because hospitalizing him on a locked ward and then communicating her concerns to the hospital had adequately protected the wife.

Applying Dr. Simon's rules for assessment of violence as shown in Table 1 of Chapter 3 yields the following violence facilitators (rated high, medium, or low): presence of motive, high to medium; absence of therapeutic relationship, high; current acute stress, medium; victim was identified and available, high; patient violent in the emergency room, high; and psychiatric diagnosis, medium. Violence inhibitors are no history of past violence, medium; rather old for first violence, medium; married, medium; employed, medium; violence not ego-syntonic, high; and no alcohol or drug abuse, medium to high.

In this case example, there are as many violence facilitators as inhibitors. In the emergency room, the facts that staff did not know this patient and that he required restraints tipped the balance toward hospitalization. On 1-year follow-up, the patient reported that he was still married, still working, and doing well. He said the clinical intervention including hospitalization had been helpful in resolving the acute crisis.

Case Example 2

The following case example illustrates an emergency room evaluation of a patient who did have an ongoing psychotherapeutic relationship.

L.J. is a 23-year-old single, unemployed Lebanese Christian man who had been hospitalized 6 months previously for psychotic depression through the emergency room. His therapist brought him to the emergency room because of her concern about the recurrence of a psychotic depression and his acute potential for violence. During the therapy hour, he had revealed to his therapist his wish to kill his mother and brother. The therapist felt threatened herself and turned to the psychiatric emergency service for assistance in assessing and treating L.J.

In the emergency room interview, the patient expressed anger and sadness around family plans to return to Lebanon. He expressed impulses to kill both his mother and younger brother, without specific plans on how he would do this. He currently lived with his mother, but his brother was overseas on an extended visit.

The patient's mental status revealed depression, psychotic symptoms of auditory hallucinations, paranoia, and ambivalence. He was able to observe these violent thoughts as "bad" and stated that he did not want to act on them and wanted help with them. He denied drug or alcohol use and any history of violence. His differential diagnosis was schizoaffective disorder versus brief reactive psychosis.

Staff invited the mother into the emergency room, and the patient told her himself about his "bad" thoughts and his desire for help with them. Mrs. J. denied any past history of violence or threats toward her by the patient and was not fearful of him. The patient showed a good response to antipsychotics in the emergency room, and a plan was made for intensive outpatient treatment. The patient received an increased dose of medication and daily visits in the psychiatric emergency room with his mother and was wait-listed for a hospital bed if his condition did not continue to improve. In addition, the subject of the son's and mother's conflict over where to live was raised, and the patient was able to express his anger at her urging him to return with her to Lebanon. The patient was hospitalized voluntarily a few days later when his psychosis worsened and his fears of his own impulses increased.

Applying Dr. Simon's rules again, variables facilitating violence are motive, low; age and sex, high; victim identified and available, high; and psychiatric diagnosis, high(?). Variables inhibiting violence are therapeutic alliance, high; other relationship, high; no substance abuse history, medium; no specific plan, high; and no history of violence, high.

In contrast to the first case example, in this case, the violence-inhibiting factors outweigh the facilitating ones. Staff were comfortable to make a plan for increased outpatient treatment rather than hospitalization. The case of L.J. illustrates the use of psychiatric emergency facilities as an extension of the relationship with a personal therapist. At 1-year follow-up there had been no violence, but L.J. had not done well. He had been hospitalized several times, his diagnosis was now schizoaffective disorder, and he was troubled by wishes to kill family members when he became psychotic. He returned to Lebanon and was lost to follow-up.

Case Example 3

The following case example illustrates that usual procedures sometimes may not sufficiently protect a potential victim. In the usual case in which a potentially violent patient is hospitalized, the emergency room staff does not warn the victim of the threat, with the reasoning that hospitalization protects the victim for the present, and it is the hospital's responsibility to assess potential violence and warn or take other appropriate action at discharge. In this case, however, because the threat was chronic, the decision was made to hospitalize and warn. Perhaps the tragic history of the Kennedy family led to particular caution in this instance.

R.T. is a 29-year-old divorced white man with schizoaffective disorder who was on Social Security disability. He suffered from chronic delusions and fantasies regarding the Kennedy family. He came voluntarily to the emergency room requesting "long-term" hospitalization, stating he was "tired of being raped and abused by everyone, especially the Kennedys." His outpatient therapist confirmed that the patient had been fighting against a decompensation over the past few weeks. He was increasingly depressed and preoccupied with his delusions regarding the Kennedys. The patient could not identify a specific member of the family at whom he was angry, nor could he describe a specific plan of dangerous behavior toward them. However, medical records revealed that the Hyannis police had arrested the patient 1 year previously for loitering around the Kennedy compound, and that he had been hospitalized. The patient had abused substances in his early 20s but denied any recent drug or alcohol use.

The psychiatrist agreed with the patient about his need for hospitalization and hospitalized him, fearing the patient was at increased risk of harming the Kennedys because of his increased psychosis. The transfer note documented the risk of harm. The psychiatrist was concerned that this was insufficient to protect the potential victims so she contacted the Hyannis police and told them about the patient, including that he was currently hospitalized. The police knew of him from his previous contact there, appreciated the psychiatrist's report, and said they would be on the alert if he should reappear.

Applying Dr. Simon's rules to this case, facilitators of violence include motive, high; psychiatric diagnosis, high; employment status, medium to low; male at the upper limit of the young age-group, medium; ambivalent about violent wishes, low; history of impulsive behavior, medium; psychiatric diagnosis, low; and history of substance abuse, low. Inhibitors of violence include therapeutic alliance, medium; no available lethal means, medium; victim unavailable, low; ambivalent about violent wishes, low; no plan, medium; no specific person threatened, high; and no recent substance abuse, low.

As in many cases, there are conflicting indicators, some suggesting that violence may be facilitated and others suggesting that it may be inhibited. This illustrates the more general point that psychiatric patients are almost always conflicted about their violent impulses. The psychiatrist who acts to help contain the violence supports the healthy side of the patient's personality against the forces of unbridled impulse expression with which the patient is struggling. In this case, the psychiatrist was concerned about the potential future exposure of the victims because of their public position. She also knew that the hospital could not be counted on to inform anyone of the patient's discharge. For that reason, she decided to inform the police herself even though there was no immediate danger. This illustrates that clinical judgment is called for in deciding how to proceed in these cases. Fulfilling the letter of the law is no substitute.

Case Example 4

The emergency room increasingly sees and evaluates a group of patients not generally seen in outpatient psychiatric treatment settings. This group consists of dangerous, character-disordered, and/or substance-abusing patients, often brought in by the police or otherwise in trouble with the law. Appelbaum has recently discussed the difficulty psychiatrists face when treating these patients, and the controversial role of psychiatry in protecting society in cases in which mental illness is not clearly involved (16,17). The psychiatric emergency service is uniquely involved with these cases, and clinicians in these settings are attempting to sort out psychiatry's responsibilities in dealing with them.

K.M. is a 55-year-old single, unemployed man who was brought to the psychiatric emergency room by the police. They were concerned about the patient's potential for violence. He had been at the mayor's office reportedly threatening to kill his own niece, Alice, because she was stealing his benefit checks and spending the money. He said he owned three guns and described each in detail. He was grossly intoxicated (alcohol level .313), with slurred speech and unsteady gait, and gave a long history of alcoholism.

According to the referring police officers, he had been arrested 1 month prior on charges of child molestation and was awaiting trial. Previous court involvements were unknown. He denied previous psychiatric contacts, although he had been in numerous detoxification centers over the years. He was allowed to remain in *the emergency room for many hours to sober up, which he did. Sober, he still insisted he would kill his niece.*

There was no clear DSM-III-R Axis I diagnosis other than alcohol abuse. He did have significant and debilitating Axis II pathology (antisocial and borderline traits). He was not under arrest. He continued to be a homicidal risk.

It is an unsettled question whether patients without Axis I disorders are committable. In a few states, the statute is broad enough to cover both Axis I and Axis II disorders. However, in most states, there is not a clear correspondence between the language of the statute and the Axes of DSM-III-R. Every practitioner should know the statutory language governing commitment and should think through his or her own position on what kinds of persons or disorders are committable.

We believe that in the state where this occurred, civil commitment ordinarily requires an Axis I disorder. The psychiatrist in this case doubted that K.M. met standards for commitment to a psychiatric facility. However, she could see no alternative way to protect the potential victim. She first breached the patient's confidentiality in an effort to warn the niece, hoping also that the niece would provide information that would help to assess the dangerousness of the situation. Unfortunately, the niece's phone was disconnected. The police went to her home but could not find her.

Applying Dr. Simon's rules, variables facilitating violence include motive, high; absence of any therapeutic alliance, high; psychiatric diagnosis, medium; situational status, medium; unemployed, medium; available guns, very high; available victim, high; and syntonic violence, high. Inhibiting factors include older age, low to medium; and lack of a specific plan, medium(?). This patient has a clear preponderance of indicators facilitating violence.

Arguably, this patient is not committable to a mental hospital because alcoholism is not a disorder that the state hospital treats. Strictly, the best course would have been to either *1)* petition the courts to commit this patient under the statute in this jurisdiction that authorizes 30-day involuntary hospitalization when there is a likelihood of serious harm by reason of alcohol or drug abuse or

2) have a witness to the threats file criminal charges and then commit the patient through the courts.

Neglecting these niceties, the emergency room psychiatrist responded appropriately. Recognizing danger, she moved to prevent harm in the only way available on the spot: involuntary hospitalization. Our hospital attorney always says, "When in doubt whether something is legal or illegal, act. Better to act and save a life and explain that in court later than not to act and have a possible tragedy and explain that in court later."

There was no follow-up. Our service never saw this patient again.

Conclusion

The *Tarasoff* decision generally reflects practices already in effect in most psychiatric emergency services. In crisis situations, when patients are seriously ill and often at their most dangerous, conservative treatment plans are necessary for the protection of the patient and the potential victims. The same professional and legal respect for patient confidentiality holds true in the emergency setting as in other clinical settings. Yet the limits of data gathering, the weaker alliance between the patient and emergency staff, and the difficulty in reliable transfer of information between facilities result in treatment plans that tend toward psychiatric hospitalization for containment and protection and/or the breaking of patient confidentiality to warn and aid in protection for potential victims. The majority of patients in the emergency room voluntarily cooperate in warning potential victims. This process can be the beginning of clinical recovery for the patient, even if it does not avert hospitalization or other restrictive alternatives.

The four case examples in this chapter have some common features. In each, the patient was hospitalized. In two cases of threatened family violence, we involved the victim in the clinical management. In both cases, we were successful in facilitating direct discussion between the patient and the potential victim. These two cases illustrate that violence is often the result of family conflict. In these cases, simple warning is not the best choice of action. Warning may protect the victim from immediate threat, but it does nothing to defuse the conflict. Discussion between the patient and the potential victim is intended to diminish family conflict and, ultimately, to help prevent violence.

In the fourth case, we tried unsuccessfully to reach K.M.'s niece. Had we reached her, we would have attempted to initiate the kind of dialogue described above. Cases such as R.T. and the Kennedys involve some unique problems. When the potential violence is based on delusional association rather than on failure to resolve realistic conflict, there is no point in imagining that any direct contact would be helpful. Rather, external controls should be brought to bear so that if the patient's internal controls are insufficient, the victim is still protected. In the court-related experience of one of us (J.C.B.), telling the patient that the police have been notified and that they are aware of the patient's concern with the victim helps to prevent violence in two ways: first, by direct police protection of the victim, and second, by giving the patient knowledge that an external authority is watching and that consequences will follow if he or she commits some antisocial or violent act, providing additional motivation for behavior control.

The four cases involve threats that were judged to have some reality. Although third parties were involved in all four cases, it was only necessary to breach the patient's confidentiality without consent in two. In the other two, the patient consented. *Tarasoff* speaks to the issue of social control of potential violence. Often, skillful clinical work leads to strategies that involve the patient voluntarily. But when this collaboration is not forthcoming, the clinician must do what is necessary to prevent violence.

References

1. Gurevitz H: *Tarasoff*: protective privilege versus public peril. Am J Psychiatry 134:289–292, 1977
2. Tarasoff v Regents of the University of California, 551 P2d 334, 131 Cal Rptr 14 (Cal Sup Ct 1976)
3. Julavits WF: Legal issues in emergency psychiatry. Psychiatr Clin North Am 6:335–345, 1983
4. Mills MJ, Sullivan G, Eth S: Protecting third parties: a decade after *Tarasoff*. Am J Psychiatry 144:68–74, 1987

5. Roth MD: *Tarasoff*: patient privacy vs. public protection. MD Med J 30:40–50, 1981
6. Roth MD, Levin LJ: Dilemma of *Tarasoff*: must physicians protect the public from their patients? Law, Medicine and Health Care June, 1983, pp 104–131
7. Kermani EJ, Drob SL: *Tarasoff* decision: a decade later dilemma still faces psychotherapists. Am J Psychotherapy 41:271–285, 1987
8. Wexler DB: Patients, therapists, and third parties: the victimological virtues of *Tarasoff*. Int J Law Psychiatry 2:1–28, 1979
9. Wulsin LR, Bursztajn H, Gutheil TG: Unexpected clinical features of the *Tarasoff* decision: the therapeutic alliance, and the "duty to warn." Am J Psychiatry 140:601–603, 1983
10. Appelbaum PS: *Tarasoff*: an update on the duty to warn. Hosp Community Psychiatry 32:14–15, 1981
11. Sadoff RL: The essence of *Tarasoff*. MD Med J 30:55, 1981
12. Appelbaum PS: *Tarasoff* and the clinician: problems in fulfilling the duty to protect. Am J Psychiatry 142:425–429, 1985
13. Bloom JD, Rogers JL: The duty to protect others from your patients—*Tarasoff* spreads to the northwest. West J Med 148:231–234, 1988
14. Gross BH, Southard MJ, Lamb HR, et al: Assessing dangerousness and responding appropriately: Hedlund expands the clinician's liability established by *Tarasoff*. J Clin Psychiatry 48:9–12, 1987
15. Jablonski v U.S., 712 F2d 391 (9th Cir 1983)
16. Appelbaum PS: Hospitalization of the dangerous patient: legal pressures and clinical responses. Bull Am Acad Psychiatry Law 12:323–329, 1984
17. Appelbaum PS: The new preventive detention: psychiatry's problematic responsibility for the control of violence. Am J Psychiatry 145:779–785, 1988

CHAPTER FIVE

The Duty to Protect in Inpatient Psychiatry

Bruce C. Gage, M.D.

The freedom needed to practice good clinical medicine seems to be dissipating. Increasing fiscal pressures and greater vulnerability to malpractice litigation often place the practitioner between diametrically opposed values. Highly publicized cases, for example, *Naidu v. Laird* (1) and *Rotman v. Mirin* (2), heighten therapist awareness of this problem. In these cases, mental health professionals were found liable when one of their patients injured a third party. Psychiatrists' inability to predict violence has been well publicized (3). Although recent studies (4,5) indicate that predictions 1–3 days before potential violence may be more reliable, the public and judiciary may hold psychiatrists accountable over longer periods. When this expectation is coupled with the emphasis on brief hospitalization and careful allocation of resources, it is easy to understand the apprehension most feel when faced with a potentially violent patient.

In this chapter, I will focus on the management of several prominent medicolegal problems encountered in the inpatient setting. The intention is to show how such issues can, and should, be woven into the treatment plan along with all other clinical considerations. Hopefully, the reader will come away with the sense that consideration of these issues, including the duty to protect, can yield good clinical results, avert third-party liability, and return a sense of clinical freedom.

The first case example approaches the familiar problem of repeatedly admitting and releasing someone who is "potentially dangerous." There is evidence that the *Tarasoff* decision has influenced admission decisions (6). Others find that, despite *Tarasoff*, admissions remain appropriate (7). There is no systematic study of discharging the violent patient in the literature. What is clear is that *Tarasoff* influences the approach to both the gate-keeping function and psychiatric treatment in general. In the context of this case example, a strategy for making discharge decisions about potentially violent patients is formulated. This strategy combines tort law and the criminal responsibility test as a tool for making decisions about whether to pursue commitment and for determining if a duty to protect is present. The second case example uses this strategy under different clinical circumstances and focuses more on its application.

The third case example examines the duty to protect within a hospital. Rossi et al. (8) has found a trend of increasing violence among patients admitted to inpatient units. Yet, there is little discussion regarding the duty to protect inpatients from each other, and this has not been considered under the rubric of *Tarasoff*. This may reflect a tacit (societal) conviction that mental patients are not citizens in the same sense as most of us. This issue is becoming more significant. Appelbaum (9) has suggested that preoccupation with third-party liability leads to an increase in the admission of character-disordered patients. These patients can be disruptive to the milieu of the psychiatric ward (10). Other observers have noted increased admission of criminals (11).

The impact of *Tarasoff* on the gatekeeping function and on constitution of the ward underscores the importance of instituting standardized treatment guidelines that specifically address the violent patient, especially with regard to the duty to protect. It is unfortunate that the preoccupation with third-party liability leads us to consider this issue not on a clinical basis, but out of self-protection. However, this should not distract us from the potential clinical utility of sound medicolegal practice. What makes this situation more perplexing is the lack of clear judicial guidelines for determining liability. Most concerning are the cases in which a doctrine of strict liability has been approached. Del Carmen (12, p. 202) described this doctrine:

> While tort is generally predicated on the concept of wrong, strict liability is based on the principle that in some cases the defendant may be held liable, although he is not charged with any moral wrongdoing, neither has he departed in any way from a reasonable standard of intent or care. Strict liability is imposed without fault and is premised on the

principle that one who innocently causes harm should pay for the damage inflicted.

Davis v. Lhim (13), *Lipari v. Sears* (14), *Jablonski v. U.S.* (15), *Naidu* (1), and possibly *Petersen v. Washington* (16) are notable examples in which this standard has been approached (17). The courts indicated that the victim foreseeably was endangered in *Davis*, as was a class of persons in *Lipari*, and that there was negligence in *Jablonski*, *Naidu*, and *Petersen*. However, these decisions are questionable, for in both instances in which "foreseeability" was invoked, there had been no specific threats. In the other three, what the court deemed negligent would be considered standard practice. *Davis* has, in fact, been overturned, but primarily because the courts found the psychiatrist immune because of his position with the state. However, the opinion also indicated there was no foreseeable victim (17).

It is unrealistic to practice assuming this form of liability. Because prediction of violence over extended periods of time is impossible, practitioners would incur enormous potential liability for nearly all discharges. Nor is the concept of negligent release sufficient. Reasonable guidelines based on traditional tort law and more mainstream cases can inform psychiatrists. Del Carmen (12) says liability may be incurred *1*) when there is abuse of discretion, gross negligence, or lack of due care; *2*) when there is foreseeability; and *3*) when there is a special relationship.

Beck's discussion (18) of these principles is discernible to the nonlawyer. In brief, the first holds the practitioner to a standard of clinical care commensurate with the practice of competent members of the pertinent professional community; the practitioner must adhere to accepted practices. In the second, "foreseeability" can be understood to mean that specific victim(s) could have been identified before the incident. The special relationship in the third can be interpreted as the patient-therapist relationship. If the three conditions enumerated above are met and are the proximate cause of injury, there is culpability. The time period over which "proximate cause" extends after discharge of the patient is not clear, the longest being five and one-half months in *Naidu*.

In response to the vicissitudes in third-party liability decisions, the American Psychiatric Association (APA) Council on Psychiatry and Law drafted a model bill for proposed legislation on the state level. A dozen states (among them, California, Maryland, Michigan, and Massachusetts) have adopted legislation similar to this model. In general, it allows a practitioner to discharge his duty to protect in warning, notifying the authorities, or hospitalizing the patient. It is important for the clinician to know the particular language in his or her jurisdiction.

Case Example 1

This case involves a man in his 40s who has had numerous hospitalizations. The most recent admissions will provide the medium for discussing the inpatient management and discharge planning for the recurrently violent patient. It is the case of a man obsessed with a woman who has spurned him. His heartache has left him with the desire to do away with the object of his yearning. The man's long-standing struggle with alcoholism complicates the situation.

B was born to a working-class family with no history of alcoholism or mental illness. The family was repeatedly disrupted. When he was 6, the children were placed in foster homes, B by himself, the other six children together. The family was reunited some 5 years later. B, with his father's help, began drinking at a young age. Throughout school, B had trouble with the law, owing in part to his drinking. He left home in his late teens, but at age 20 returned "to take care of [his] mother" after the death of his father.

B's first two admissions followed his mother's death 17 years ago; heavy drink was his solace. His diagnoses were alcoholism and passive-aggressive personality disorder.

Shortly after discharge, he married. After the birth of his first child, he maintained sobriety without support programs and worked fairly steadily. He and his wife separated 6 years ago. Soon after the separation, his life crumbled. He drank heavily and lost his job and health insurance.

Five years ago, he was admitted with suicidal ideation and had a concomitant desire to kill his wife. This began the series of hospitalizations pertinent to the current topic.

*After detoxification, he resumed blaming his wife for his sit-
uation. He declared his intention to "kill [his] wife sober or not."
B revealed that he had in fact assaulted his wife. The psychiatrist
contacted the district attorney, who, at the psychiatrist's suggestion,
warned B's wife of her husband's dangerousness and urged her to
press charges. She chose not to press charges but did obtain a restraining order. The psychiatrist wrote a note detailing this and
added that "[B] is not now, and has not been during this admission,
mentally ill." It was further documented that B understood the
wrongfulness of murder. But as he still contemplated murder, could
he be released?*

Here we look into the abyss of what Appelbaum has so aptly
designated "the new preventive detention" (6). This trend resulted
from the shift to a dangerousness standard in commitment laws
(9,19). A recent Colorado court stated:

> . . . the psychiatrist has a legal duty . . . to determine whether
> the patient has a propensity for violence and would thereby present
> an unreasonable risk of serious bodily harm to others if released from
> the involuntary commitment, and, further, that . . . the psychiatrist
> may be required to take reasonable precautions to protect the public
> from the danger created by the release of the involuntarily committed
> patient, including the giving of due consideration to extending the term
> of the patient's commitment or to placing appropriate conditions and
> restrictions on the patient's release. (20, p. 1201)

The problem here is that the psychiatrist is expected to protect not
specific victims, but the public at large, and, further, from any
patient who has a *propensity* for violence. What makes this even
more viscous is that judicial precedent, via *Currie v. U.S.* (21),
indicates that psychosis is not a prerequisite for commitment, although this holding was later overturned (22). Nearly any angry
soul who is intoxicated or has a possible DSM-III-R Axis II diagnosis could be construed to fall within these bounds.

Appelbaum suggests that the best way for the profession to
avoid this treacherous position is by not allowing it to become the
standard of care (6). Only those character-disordered patients who
can gain *therapeutic* benefit should be hospitalized. The upshot of
this is that admission can be justified for character-disordered pa-

tients with acute decompensations, but not for those with chronic characterologic violence. Work by Segal et al. (23) suggests this battle is being won. Their research indicates that despite utilization of "danger to others" as a criterion for commitment, relatively few character-disordered patients entered the hospital by this route. In fact, most of those admitted for danger to others were also severely mentally ill. Attention to Appelbaum's admonition will help maintain this finding and preserve the therapeutic mission of inpatient units.

This principle can also be applied to the discharge of such patients. Once the acute situation is resolved, discharge can proceed despite the fact that these patients are likely to be violent again. In the case of the substance abuser, a similar approach can be used. Criminal law has long held that intoxication during commission of a crime is not in itself grounds for exculpation (24,25). Because substance abusers with no mental illness are responsible for their behavior, they need not be kept in the hospital solely to prevent violence associated with intoxication. Unfortunately, some states have commitment laws that provide for commitment of persons solely on the basis of intoxication. Practitioners in these regions may have to detain these patients until sober, but once sober, they can be discharged.

Patients with psychoses present a different problem: the psychosis may interfere with their judgment. When such patients commit violent acts, there is a greater likelihood that the psychiatrist will incur third-party liability. For this reason, the psychiatrist should undertake an evaluation based on the legal concept of criminal responsibility before discharging any potentially violent patient. Only the courts can determine whether someone can be held criminally responsible for their actions. The application of this test in the clinical setting is by no means legally binding and is intended only as a problem-solving tool.

To be held criminally responsible, persons must be able both to appreciate the wrongfulness of their actions and to conform their conduct to the requirements of the law (i.e., be "culpable"). Although character-disordered patients appreciate wrongfulness and have the ability to conform their conduct, they may choose otherwise and are thus culpable. Those with psychoses, affective disorders, and other Axis I disorders may not be culpable on one or both grounds.

This test is more clinically useful than the usual formula: failure to hospitalize would create a likelihood of serious harm by reason of mental illness. There are many types of mentally ill and character-disordered patients who are known to be likely to be violent even at their best and thus always present a likelihood of serious harm and could never be comfortably discharged with this criterion. The "criminal responsibility test" provides more specific criteria that address the degree to which someone is both in control of his or her impulses and understands societal bounds as demarcated by the law. So although someone may be impulsive and likely to be involved in violence, he or she can still be released if able to control his or her impulses, even though more likely than others to be violent over time. Perhaps more importantly, this test moves the focus of accountability from the therapist to the patient: instead of the therapist deciding whether it is likely that the patient will do harm, the therapist decides only whether the patient is able to resist impulses, placing the burden of responsibility more on the patient. This is almost always more therapeutic as well.

Combining the preceding analysis with the foreseeability criterion of tort law yields the following four decision categories:

1. If, in the opinion of the psychiatrist, the patient would be considered culpable (should anything happen) and there is no foreseeable victim, discharge can be based on an assessment of the benefit of continued hospitalization, even if the patient is potentially violent.
2. If the patient would be culpable and there is a foreseeable victim, then the duty to protect applies. However, the patient can be discharged after appropriate attention to the duty to protect, such as warning the potential victim and contacting the pertinent police department.
3. For those patients considered potentially violent and who would not be held culpable but there is no foreseeable victim, commitment should be strongly considered. The more closely the potential for violence is related to mental illness, e.g., in hal-

lucinations or delusions, the more strongly commitment should be considered.

4. If there is a foreseeable victim and the patient would not be held culpable, commitment is indicated.

In the last two categories, if the situation is unchanged after appropriate treatment, two courses are available: recommitment or reintegration into the community with careful attention to the duty to protect. The courts are aware of the potential risks inherent in the most skillful reintegration and will not find negligence solely because of a bad outcome (26,27). Some authors recommend use of a committee to review difficult discharges (28). This is reasonable but creates a standard of care that uses much needed resources. Good documentation and judicious consultation are adequate.

B was released as it had been clearly documented that his propensity to violence was not the result of mental illness. This is an instance of category 2 as delineated above. Although there is a "foreseeable victim," the foreseeable victim had been amply advised, meeting the duty to protect aspect of this category. And although a special relationship exists, the lack of a mental illness precludes involuntary hospitalization. The psychiatrist thus does not have sufficient control to be held liable. In addition, as further hospitalization was not clinically indicated, discharge was warranted on this basis as well. It is important to note that these points were specifically addressed by the team and documented in the chart, showing that "due care" was taken.

Soon B was entrenched in street living. He began to present in the emergency room with injuries incurred in fights but was usually not admitted. Two years ago, he presented to the psychiatric emergency room and there attempted to hang himself. Although there was no evidence of psychosis or affective disorder, he was clearly deteriorating and was still obsessed with his estranged wife. Therefore, he was admitted for an acute decompensation. He was placed on one-to-one observation, and a physician's order was written: "notify pt's wife and her local police if B elopes." Although writing such an order does not alone satisfy the physician's obligation to the potential victim, it serves to alert the staff and it shows a good-faith effort. B managed a graceful discharge after a short stay for detoxification. This time it was not necessary to contact his wife at the time of discharge because B had made it clear that he did not intend to harm her. Further, his cooperation with treatment demonstrated his good intentions.

The staff began to wonder whether some of his behavior represented his way of asking for help. They noted that since the initiation of the restraining order, there had been only threats. Thus, it seemed that the external control afforded by the restraining order had helped curb his acting out toward his wife. And further, although the ostensible target of his threats was the same, the goal was shifting from reclamation of his wife to hospital admission—a transformation of dependence needs. During his next stay, the staff strongly recommended halfway house placement. B was resistant, substantiating the view that there was a growing institutional dependence.

The preceding is important for two reasons: *1*) The use of external controls can be as powerful outside the hospital as inside. *2*) These controls can help effect dynamic change if properly employed. These are the principles allowing the integration of good clinical practice and medicolegal prudence.

The current admission followed several instances of harassing his wife in violation of the restraining order. B was more vituperative than usual and continued to threaten that he really would kill his wife. When told of the continued intention to warn his wife, he responded: "Fine, it's been done three times already."

Because of the apparent inadequacy of the extant controls, the psychiatrist obtained a forensic consultation. The consultant felt there was some evidence that B was suffering from a major depression and might be bipolar. As such, there was a possibility that his "potential dangerousness" derived from a mental illness amenable to inpatient treatment. This shifted B to category 4—not culpable and a foreseeable victim. The consultant recommended further hospitalization and trials of appropriate medications. A meeting with the wife, the police, and a suitable social service agency was also suggested. Various prospects for her protection could be proffered, including relocation and seeking additional police aid.

This moves beyond a mere warning. When warnings, restraining orders, and similar "first-line" mechanisms have been employed and the situation continues to escalate, such additional steps are indicated. The patient may feel that existing controls are impotent, as in this case when the patient defiantly responds that warnings have already been given. These steps inform all parties that the relative danger has increased.

B became increasingly uncooperative and threatened escape. Because of B's continued dangerousness and the possibility that his condition was treatable (and related to his dangerousness), the psychiatrist sought commitment; this is the appropriate course for a patient in category 4. It was granted. He was begun on an antidepressant and neuroleptic, but B soon began to refuse medication. Medication was discontinued and, without his consent, could only be given during emergencies. The staff felt B was competent to make decisions about medications, so judicial permission to treat was not sought. B agreed to a trial of lithium, but it yielded no benefit.

When patients refuse medication and remain potentially dangerous secondary to mental illness, commitment is indicated. Difficulty arises when these patients are competent to make medication decisions, and commitment statutes do not allow the psychiatrist to give medications involuntarily. In such instances, if milieu, psychotherapy, and other techniques do not result in remission, the psychiatrist must seek permission to treat, often from the courts. Appelbaum (29) provides a detailed discussion of various models of treatment refusal and their implications in practice. If permission to treat is not granted, the patient must be detained in the hospital until released by the courts or until there is sufficient improvement to allow discharge.

Earlier, B had learned that his wife had begun divorce proceedings. Her plan resulted, in part, from the aforementioned meeting. Although this might have caused B's recent distress, the ambiguity of separation almost certainly contributed to his previous deterioration. Again, what was originally a Tarasoff intervention yielded profits in other realms.

To support him through the divorce, the staff allowed B to stay in the hospital. The depressive symptoms abated, and he joined a work program. A lawyer was secured, and B attended the divorce proceedings. He did not act out in court. His commitment expired but he chose to stay in the hospital through the divorce.

To pursue halfway house placement, community passes had to be arranged. His wife was informed of each pass. Because of his lack of motivation in this direction, the staff began to discuss discharging B. The forensic consultant returned and, in discussion with senior staff, came to the conclusion that there was no evidence of depression. Further history had not revealed any other Axis I illness. B was alcoholic and character disordered. His performance in court clearly demonstrated his ability to resist the still recurring impulse to harm his wife. Combining this with his appreciation of the wrongfulness of murder, he clearly meets the criteria for culpability and can be returned to category 2.

Though he had made no recent threats to harm his wife, a warning about discharge was clearly in order. There are several reasons for this. First, with the finalization of the divorce, any hope of reconciliation was dashed and it was not clear how B would respond to the outcome he had feared for so long. Second, his dubious commitment to treatment portended continued maladaptive functioning. Third, there had been a clear precedent set during this hospitalization. With the patient present, the therapist telephoned both the police and B's wife. He informed them of B's discharge and history of threats and assaultiveness. He also told them that, after careful evaluation, the staff felt that B was clearly responsible for his actions and subject to criminal prosecution should anything happen.

At 3-year follow-up, B has not returned to the hospital. His ex-wife called once 18 months after his discharge to ask how to get B back in treatment but indicated no other problems.

Case Example 2

C is a 36-year-old man with a diagnosis of chronic paranoid schizophrenia. He has had numerous hospitalizations, many following assaults in the community. Before this hospitalization, he had damaged a stranger's car with a rake while the car was at a stoplight. C believed the stranger was "staking [him] out." He exhibited signs of a thought disorder but denied hallucinations and thought control. There was no evidence of affective disorder. Further inquiry revealed that C believed himself to be an undercover narcotics agent who was in jeopardy of being discovered and killed by drug dealers. When asked if there was a specific person or group of people who were trying to uncover his identity, he responded in the negative. He also denied homicidal ideation toward any particular person(s). However, C also stated that he would be able to identify "a dealer" and would take "whatever steps are necessary" to protect himself. He thought he might find these people "hanging out in the street" near his residence.

We undertook an evaluation based on the criminal responsibility test. C understood that murder and assault were crimes and that he could go to jail if found guilty. He also felt that such acts were "wrong" and should be punished. While on the ward, C was generally a model patient, addressing staff as "sir" and helping other patients. He occasionally yelled at other patients but could be calmed by verbal means and would often apologize when in the wrong. It was clear that he had the ability to appreciate the wrongfulness of murder and assault, thereby satisfying the first criterion of culpability.

C was compliant with medication and felt that he needed it to "keep [his] thinking clear" and, in fact, showed improvement in his thought disorder. However, he had no insight into his delusional system and continued to insist on the veracity of his undercover identity. In this capacity, C indicated he would have no compunction about killing someone of "the criminal element." Because of his delusional beliefs about himself and potential victims, he might not be able to conform his conduct to the requirements of the law. In his mind, he would not be committing murder but would be upholding the law. Our opinion was that he did not satisfy the criteria of criminal responsibility and would not be held culpable.

Here is a patient in category 3: he is potentially violent and would not be held culpable, but there is no readily identifiable foreseeable victim. As such, our decision tree indicated that we should strongly consider commitment. Because there was a history of past and recent violence that was directly related to his mental illness, we initiated commitment proceedings. At a probable cause hearing, the commitment was upheld. C subsequently pursued a writ of habeas corpus. At the hearing, he denied homicidal and

*destructive intent and ideation. The writ was granted, and C had
to be released. Concern about his continued violence potential led
us to call the police department in C's community and his landlady
and inform them of our concern, thereby fulfilling our duty to
protect in this jurisdiction.*

*Three weeks later, he returned after having assaulted another
stranger for the same reason.*

Case Example 3

*D is a 31-year-old woman who has been residing voluntarily
in a state hospital for 7 years. When at her best, she is a leader on
the ward, even acting as mediator in disputes. At her worst, she is
wildly out of control. She acts out sexually, incites other patients,
and can be seriously assaultive.*

*D came from a poor family and grew up in the inner city where
mastery of the art of street combat was essential. She learned the
importance of devoted allies on the one hand, and total commitment
to battle on the other. This polar view of life was echoed in her
family life. She had an identical twin who was favored by her father,
D by her mother. The parents eventually divorced, and D was
scapegoated by her twin and at times by her mother. Her developmental history is notable for fire setting and some acting out and
drug abuse in high school. After graduation, she found employment
as a secretary. She later began to steal and was convicted of larceny.
There was no guilt, only shame at being caught; she felt entitled
to some material advantages.*

*D's first hospitalizations, beginning at age 22, were brief. She
would present acutely manic without psychosis. Haloperidol was
effective in controlling her mania, but after discharge, she would
soon stop taking medications and decompensate. This cycle was
repeated several times in the ensuing year.*

*Psychological testing revealed a person whose inner world was
the entire world, who was remote from understanding the needs of
others, and who showed sudden shifts in mood. Impulse control
was constantly in jeopardy.*

*Later, after an overdose, she was hospitalized for over a year.
Restraint and seclusion were frequent. She finally agreed to a trial
of lithium and responded well. After discharge, she was stable for*

9 months but then stopped her medication, became manic, and lost her placement.

When she returned to the hospital, it was to stay. Being a permanent resident of the hospital changed the nature of her relationship with staff and other patients. Without the goal of discharge, good behavior was no longer essential. Over this period, it became clear that she suffered from rapid-cycling bipolar affective disorder. Her cycling could be controlled by lithium but D often chose not to take her medications. Between episodes, she was euthymic but continued to act out periodically. This impulsivity differed from her manic behavior in that it was clearly done with a purpose in mind or in response to some perceived slight or unmet expectation.

As she was a voluntary patient, several issues arose: 1) Was continued hospitalization wise or indicated? 2) Should she have a guardian? 3) What leverage was available that could be both legally and ethically employed?

When remission of Axis I symptoms reveals a patient who has violent proclivities of character, Gutheil and Appelbaum (30) have pointed out the importance of balancing the patient's potential for violence out of the hospital, and the attendant danger to the citizenry and possible third-party liability, with the disruption caused to the ward by the violent (character-disordered) patient. In the past, such patients who became disruptive were discharged without great concern. Although it may at times be distasteful to have to pursue such a balance, the courts have made it clear that we must. Many feel this will eventuate in countertherapeutic practice. However, struggling with the rules of society is often key to a patient's recovery, and what better way to approach this than through accountability for one's actions? The therapist, as a proactive agent in the patient's life, must (perhaps inherently) participate in this.

Because D decompensated so rapidly in the community, it seemed clear that she should stay, regardless of the impact on the milieu. Because she was competent when compensated, it was doubtful that the courts would grant guardianship. Finally, the only leverage available was to rescind her privileges when she broke ward rules or was a danger to self or others. However, it was not legal or ethical to coerce her into taking medications by making privileges contingent on compliance; if competent to make decisions about treatment, it is a patient's right to refuse.

This remained the state of affairs until several years later when D was found to be positive for antibodies to the human immunodeficiency virus (HIV). D now presented a new kind of danger to the community. Two new issues arose: Who can we tell? How has our duty to protect changed, if at all?

Clearly, this scenario is becoming more common. Until legislatures create new laws specifically addressing the HIV-positive patient (e.g., as has happened in Florida and California) or, less desirably, the judiciary rules on such cases, mental health professionals must assume that the duty to protect applies. Some authors contend that the duty to protect may supersede state laws forbidding disclosure in some instances, owing to ethical as well as legal considerations (31). APA has published two policy statements that are useful but provide only very general recommendations (32,33). These issues are discussed at length in Chapter 8. In addition, there are a number of extant medicolegal tools and precedents that can inform the practitioner treating the HIV-positive patient.

What makes the dangerous inpatient (not just the HIV-positive patient) difficult to manage is that each patient can only be dealt with in the context of a particular clinical situation. The APA policy statements and *Tarasoff* serve only as guidelines that must be weighed against the backdrop of good clinical and ethical practice. The balance between confidentiality and the duty to protect was discussed at length by Beck (34). One clear tenet that emerges is the necessity to involve the patient in the discussion. This resonates with the above contention regarding patients' accountability, that is, it conveys the idea that the patient has at least played a part in creating the situation and must be involved in its resolution.

We began by discussing the results and implications of the HIV test with D. She assured us that she would not have sex with other patients. Knowing this was unlikely, we asked her to use condoms and instructed her in their use. D elected not to tell other patients but was informed that some staff would need to know because of the medical problems associated with HIV. Other staff would be told that she was on body-fluid precautions. This is consistent with the APA policy statement.

A period of calm and improved communication ensued during which she took her medications. This period came to an end after 6 months. She resumed her pattern of intermittent medication compliance and had several brief hypomanic episodes. On one occasion, she threatened to give AIDS to a staff member. Concern leapt when she was discovered in bed with a male patient. The staff who reviewed her case found that D would discontinue her medications following object loss or disappointment, seeming to use her illness as retribution. This was in keeping with her developmental history and psychological testing. In short, it was apparent that this reflected characterologic features more than her affective disorder; there was no recourse but to use the behavioral means at our disposal and to help her see the pattern.

We considered an administrative discharge but knew that she would soon return, and that in the interim, there was a high likelihood that she would have unprotected intercourse. Although there may not have been foreseeable victims, it was unethical to place the public at risk when it was virtually certain she would return in the near future. Because there is no specific threat or foreseeable victim, this is not an application of "Tarasoff thinking"; it is more akin to the notion of negligent release. But it is important to remember that third-party liability might be incurred on this basis as well (e.g., as in Perreira v. State of Colorado, et al. [20]). *Use of the criminal responsibility test at this point would place her in category 1 (considered culpable but with no foreseeable victim), and discharge would not be unthinkable. However, the likelihood of a rapid decompensation into mania on discharge suggests that D should be considered to be in category 3 (not culpable with no foreseeable victim), and thus continued hospitalization should be strongly considered.*

It is reasonable to assert that an HIV-positive patient constitutes a *potential* danger to others similar to that posed by a patient with a deadly weapon. This amplifies the duty to protect. With several cases pending involving the question of whether HIV can be used as a weapon, this seems a prudent stance to take on legal as well as ethical grounds. It is possible to remove a weapon from someone voluntarily or, with judicial assistance, involuntarily (and this should be done more regularly). The infeasibility of this with AIDS is problematic and there is no clear solution.

Opinion was divided about whether to tell other patients about the danger of sexual relations with D. As not all were at risk, we felt that it would constitute a breach of confidentiality to inform the whole community; there was inadequate justification (i.e., the whole community did not need to be protected). We considered telling only those deemed to be at risk, but another obstacle presented itself: Would a mere warning adequately protect the potential victims? Some were clearly unable to make use of the information. Meanwhile, the staff began to educate the ward about AIDS. This still left those who were "incompetent to be warned." Here we came up against both the limitations of the law and of the clinical setting. No viable mode of protection offered itself. The only effective solution would be to isolate D, a solution all abhorred. In situations where constant observation is possible, this can be utilized if there is an acute condition that can be expected to remit.

After her sister's psychiatric admission during a pregnancy, D left the hospital against medical advice and stopped her medications. She returned hypomanic and her behavior quickly escalated. Angry at a staff member, she threatened to kill him and, minutes later, attacked him with menstrual blood on her hands, screaming, "I'll give you AIDS." Her attack succeeded as her scratch broke the skin. After a violent struggle, made worse by people's fear, she was restrained. The next morning, she was in restraints and still out of control. She tried to bite anyone who approached. D was unrecognizable. Now the question of when to remove the restraints arose. Though she had improved with medications, it was by no means certain that she would not remain assaultive. This would not have been such a problem were it not for the potential transmission of HIV. Because of this episode and her recent sexual behavior, our duty to protect was highlighted in a way that did not previously exist. We sought immediate guardianship.

Many will decry this as discriminatory, but the operative principle here is the protection of foreseeable victims of (serious) violence.

There are two primary reasons for involving the judicial system in situations in which there is significant risk of serious harm. First, it shows that this form of external control was at least attempted. Second, a course of treatment somewhat outside the ordinary may be anticipated. If guardianship is granted, the courts will oversee the treatment from the outset, providing input and greater freedom. The freedom does not stem solely from obtaining the right to treat against the patient's will, but also from dissolution of the tendency to second-guess oneself about preserving patients' rights. This derives from alleviating the fear of our own retribution: the clinician no longer has to assume complete responsibility for protecting the patient's rights. The court, an institution at least as powerful as medicine, does just that. This provides an opportunity for consistency and firm limits that may not otherwise exist when, as in this case, the treatment oscillates between no treatment and responses to behavior. This is a vital aspect of guardianship that is often overshadowed by the right to give medications against a patient's will. Unfortunately, it is also frequently overlooked or forgotten when formulating treatment plans and deciding when to pursue guardianship.

Although a similar patient who did not present such significant risk of serious harm might have been released from restraints by this time, the situation demanded greater conservatism. D remained in four-point restraints for another day. Until then, D expressed no remorse or concern and, worse, would give no assurance that she would not act similarly. She insisted that her attack was warranted because a belonging had been stolen from her. In fact, she had stolen the belonging. She apologized to the victim but maintained her position that she was the injured party. She tendered her apology only because the victim was not the alleged thief. With her agreement, she was released from restraints and placed in a restraining jacket. Her behavior remained calm. We told her she was doing well but that we did not want to jeopardize her progress by moving too quickly; if a similar episode occurred, there would be similar repercussions, an eventuality nobody wanted. The staff made it clear that the other patients and staff had a right to be, and feel, safe.

*The assault victim pressed charges (a practice we strongly en-
courage) in part to communicate to D that she would be held accountable for her behavior and, more importantly, to express our
belief that she could be a responsible person—a citizen. Soon she
began to talk about returning to the regular ward and day treatment. Since all knew of her medical condition, by way of her im-
promptu revelation, confidentiality was no longer at issue. What
remained were the powerful feelings engendered by her actions. As
D spent some time on the ward in her restraining jacket, all were
able to see her in safety. For her protection, nursing provided one-
to-one observation. Her behavior and demeanor continued to be
exemplary, and there was a rising sentiment in both staff and patients to get D out of this terrible device. This continued to build
until there was a clear mandate; we yielded. D was aware of this
process and was visibly touched, leading to her reconciliation with
many. This reversal of sentiment was critical to her reincorporation
into the community and may not have been possible without the
consistency permitted by the guardianship.*

*The psychiatrist had apprised the courts of the treatment as it
progressed. Now the temporary guardianship was to expire, and we
elected to pursue permanent status, though we thought it might be
denied. Here again, we involved D in the process. She knew it was
her right to contest the guardianship. We told D that however things
turned out she could stay, and, assuming her constructive behavior
continued, she would be able to return to her day program. D elected
not to contest. Several weeks later, she returned to her day program.*

*One year later, she is becoming increasingly involved in re-
habilitative programs, and there have been no further assaults. She
remains one of the ward leaders.*

Discussion

The essence of this chapter can be distilled to three key points.
First, although the determination of liability is under the purview
of the legal system, it is our duty and privilege to set standards for
the delivery of good care. Clearly, the capacity to regulate admissions and discharges determines the constitution of inpatient wards
and, a fortiori, the quality of care that can be delivered. Setting

universally employed clinical standards that respect the ideal of treatment, rather than attempting to prevent crime, will check the advance of "the new preventive detention."

Second, the problem of third-party liability with regard to discharge, although sticky, is not insurmountable. The psychiatrist must pay careful attention to the criteria of tort law: foreseeability, negligent release (due care), and the special relationship (presence of sufficient control). Assessment of the two branches of criminal responsibility—appreciation of wrongfulness and ability to conform conduct to the code of the law—aids in the determination of the clinician's responsibility when faced with a potentially violent patient. It provides helpful indicators of whether the potential for violence is due to the type of mental illness that reduces culpability and whether there is current risk. Combining this evaluation with the foreseeability criterion yields the four decision categories presented earlier. If the practitioner also has a special relationship to the patient, as is always the case on an inpatient unit, then he or she should adhere to the dictates of these categories. However, these categories are only tools and should not be rigidly applied. D could have been released as a category 1 patient, but the team knew she would decompensate virtually immediately. Her discharge would thus have been a negligent release with the attendant liability—legal and ethical.

Third, the law does not dictate our practice; it admonishes us to stay within certain bounds. These bounds also provide us with several useful tools. In this chapter, I explored the use of the duty to protect alongside traditional interventions such as commitment, guardianship, and criminal proceedings. Incorporation of these modalities into clinical practice not only averts third-party liability but, used creatively, can enhance the outcome of treatment.

References

1. Naidu v Laird, 539 A2d 1064 (Del Supr 1988)
2. Rotman v Mirin, Middlesex Sup Court No 881562 (1988)
3. Monahan J: The clinical prediction of violent behavior (DHHS Publ No ADM-81-921). Rockville, MD, National Institute of Mental Health, 1981
4. McNeil DE, Binder RL: Predictive validity of judgments of danger-

ousness in emergency civil commitment. Am J Psychiatry 144:197–200, 1987

5. Beck JC, Bonnar J: Emergency civil commitment: predicting hospital violence from behavior in the community. Psychiatry and Law 16:379–388, 1988

6. Appelbaum PS: The new preventive detention: psychiatry's problematic responsibility for the control of violence. Am J Psychiatry 145:779–785, 1988

7. Segal SP, Watson MA, Goldfinger SM, et al: Civil commitment in the psychiatric emergency room: III. Arch Gen Psychiatry 45:759–763, 1988

8. Rossi AM, Jacobs M, Monteleone M, et al: Violent or fear-inducing behavior associated with hospital admission. Hosp Community Psychiatry 36:643–647, 1985

9. Appelbaum PS: Hospitalization of the dangerous patient: legal pressures and clinical responses. Bull Am Acad Psychiatry Law 12:323–329, 1984

10. Johansen KH: The impact of patients with chronic character pathology on a hospital inpatient unit. Hosp Community Psychiatry 34:842–846, 1983

11. Steadman JH, Cocozza JJ, Melick ME: Explaining the increased arrest rate among mental patients: the changing clientele of state hospitals. Am J Psychiatry 135:816–820, 1978

12. Del Carmen RV: Civil liabilities of government psychotherapists and agencies for the release of the mentally ill. Journal of Psychiatry and Law 12:183–213, 1984

13. Davis v Lhim, 335 NW2d 481, 124 (Mich App 291 1983)

14. Lipari v Sears, 497 FSupp 185 (D Neb 1980)

15. Jablonski v U.S., 712 F2d 391 (9th Cir 1983)

16. Petersen v Washington, 671 P2d 230, 100 (Wash 2d 421 1983)

17. Beck JC: Canon v Thumudo. American Academy of Psychiatry and the Law Newsletter 13:23–25, 1988

18. Beck JC: The psychotherapist and the violent patient: recent case law, in The Potentially Violent Patient and the Tarasoff Decision in Psychiatric Practice. Edited by Beck JC. Washington, DC, American Psychiatric Press, 1985, pp 9–34

19. Mestrovic SG, Cook JA: The dangerousness standard: what is it and how is it used? Int J Psychiatry Law 8:443–469, 1986

20. Perreira v State of Colorado et al, 768 P2d 1198 (Colo Ct App 1987)

21. Currie v U.S., FSupp 1074 (MD NC 1986)

22. Currie v U.S. v International Business Machines, 836 F2d 209 (4th Cir 1987)

23. Segal SP, Watson MA, Goldfinger SM, et al: Civil commitment in the psychiatric emergency room: II. Arch Gen Psychiatry 45:753–758, 1988
24. The Model Penal Code of the American Law Institute, § 2.08, 1962
25. Kane v U.S., 399 F2d 247, 250 (2d Cir 1972)
26. Parry J: The civil-criminal dichotomy in insanity commitment and release proceedings: Hinkley and other matters. Mental and Physical Disability Law Reporter 11:218–223, 1987
27. Taig v NY, 241 NYS2d 495 (1963)
28. Travin S, Bluestone H: Discharging the violent psychiatric patient. J Forensic Sci 32:999–1008, 1987
29. Appelbaum PS: The right to refuse treatment with antipsychotic medications: retrospect and prospect. Am J Psychiatry 145:413–419, 1988
30. Gutheil TG, Appelbaum PS: Clinical Handbook of Psychiatry and the Law. New York, McGraw-Hill, 1982, pp 127–129
31. Mills M, Wofsy CB, Mills J: The acquired immunodeficiency syndrome: infection control and public law. N Engl J Med 314:931–936, 1986
32. American Psychiatric Association: AIDS policy: Guidelines for inpatient psychiatric units. Am J Psychiatry 145:542, 1988
33. American Psychiatric Association: AIDS policy: Confidentiality and disclosure. Am J Psychiatry 145:541, 1988
34. Beck JC: A clinical survey of Tarasoff experience, in The Potentially Violent Patient and the Tarasoff Decision in Psychiatric Practice. Edited by Beck JC. Washington, DC, American Psychiatric Press, 1985, pp 59–82

CHAPTER SIX

Managing Risk and Confidentiality in Clinical Encounters With Children and Families

Richard Barnum, M.D.

Therapists dealing with children and families face many difficult situations involving potential danger, either to their patients or to others. Often, the therapist's ordinary obligation to keep communications from patients confidential is disrupted by other obligations that may be more compelling. Understanding the nature of these various obligations can be difficult. Applying them to specific clinical problems, and figuring out how to act to achieve the best balance among competing obligations, can be very challenging indeed.

The most-often discussed situations of potential danger involving children are those in which the child appears to be in danger as a result of abuse or neglect (1). However, problems of managing confidential communications in potentially dangerous circumstances arise in a variety of other situations as well.

In this chapter, I explore the issues of therapist obligation in each of these situations. I define circumstances for the mental health clinician, based on who the clinician's patient is, who the potential victim is, and to whom the clinician owes what duties. I describe legal, regulatory, and systems contexts in which actions can be taken or not taken. Finally, I briefly address some of the ethical and practical problems these situations can present for clinicians working with children and families, with case examples for illustration.

Table 1.   Child psychiatry encounters involving risk

	Victim	Perpetrator
Child patient	The child patient exposed to harm, usually definable as abuse or neglect, with exceptions. If abuse or neglect, should be reported. Other protective measures may be taken, whether risk due to abuse/neglect or not.	The child patient putting others at risk creates a *Tarasoff* obligation for the therapist. This can be met by reporting, if victim is a child, but other measures usually called for as well, both to protect victim and to further long-range interests of child-patient perpetrator.
Adult patient	An adult patient being victimized by a child creates no special legal obligation for the adult's therapist, other than to advocate appropriately with the adult for his or her safety and for help for the child. Pay attention to whether child also victimized.	The adult patient victimizing a child creates a *Tarasoff* obligation and specific obligations to report. These are independent and meeting one obligation does not discharge the other. This situation creates the clearest ethical conflicts, especially if standards of definition or impacts of intervention differ.

Situations

Any situation involving clinical evaluation or treatment in which issues of potential danger arise involving children can be described in terms of whether the patient is a child or an adult, and whether the patient is the person at risk or the likely perpetrator. These two categorizations interact to form four conditions, as shown in Table 1.

Child Patient as Victim

Most situations in which a child patient is exposed to harm are a result of abuse or neglect, usually by a parent, other family member, or school or other institutional setting. If the harm is due to abuse or neglect, then the therapist has a straightforward obligation to report the situation to a child protection or law enforcement agency. The specifics of this requirement will be explored further later in this chapter. Regardless of whether the harm is related to abuse, the therapist may also have an obligation to take some action to protect the patient beyond simple reporting. This obligation is not to a third party, but rather to the patient. It may be implicit in the duty of care that a psychiatrist owes to a child patient (2,3). Actions that might fulfill this obligation would include clinical intervention with a family or institution to change risky situations for a child, or advocating with the child and family to obtain police or other protection from the source of harm.

Adult Patient as Victim

When an adult patient faces harm at the hands of a child who is not a patient, in general, the therapist has no special obligation to act outside the therapeutic relationship to protect the patient. Within the relationship, the therapist owes the patient attention to his or her condition of victimization and may try to help the patient to improve this condition according to the therapeutic contract. This help might include advocacy for the patient seeking protection, and encouragement for the patient to seek special attention for the child, especially if the child perpetrator is the patient's own child. Regardless of whether the perpetrator is the patient's child, this special attention should include consideration of bringing appropriate legal action against the child, whether as a delinquent or a child in need of services (status offender), or through civil domestic violence action to bring a restraining order against the child.

Child Patient as Perpetrator

When a child patient appears to be putting others at risk, the child's therapist has the same *Tarasoff* obligation he or she would have if the patient were an adult. The issue here is the obligation to a third party at risk; if such a risk exists, then the obligation exists, regardless of what kind of patient is posing the risk. If the third party is also a child, then the therapist may also be obliged to report the situation as child abuse.

Tarasoff protection can be afforded in the same ways as with adults, such as warning the victim, committing the patient, enlisting the action of police and courts, or anything else that can reasonably be expected to succeed in protecting the victim (4–6). The potential harm may be reportable as child abuse if the victim is a child. If it is, and reporting the abuse appears sufficient to protect the victim (e.g., by removing the victim from proximity to the perpetrator), then the therapist can meet the *Tarasoff* obligation adequately simply by reporting. Whether the therapist still has other obligations will be explored below.

Adult Patient as Perpetrator

When an adult patient puts a child at risk, the same *Tarasoff* obligation to protect exists as for any other type of potential victim. In most situations, the harm posed by the adult will be definable as abuse or neglect and will also therefore require a child abuse report. As above, if reporting can be expected to protect the child, then reporting is sufficient to discharge the *Tarasoff* obligation. If the harm is not defined as abuse, or if reporting cannot reasonably be expected to protect the child, then the therapist must pursue other measures to provide protection. Even if the therapist takes appropriate and effective measures to protect the child from the adult patient, he or she also must report the child abuse if such reporting is required by local statutes.

This framework presents a general picture of the issues involved in the area of violence and therapist obligations in child psychiatry. It indicates that four different principles apply in understanding these obligations. The simplest is that of confidentiality. Another is the *Tarasoff* duty to protect third parties threatened by patients. A third, related to this, is a potential obligation to act to protect a patient as part of providing care and treatment. The fourth stems from statutory requirements to report child abuse.

Duties of confidentiality and protection of third parties and to provide care and treatment are not different in principle when applied to work with children and families than to work with individual adult patients, though they may sometimes be applied differently. However, the child abuse reporting obligation is quite different and raises many complex questions about what is actually required of whom, when, where, and with what consequences (1). To develop a clearer understanding of these special issues, we need to look more closely at child abuse reporting statutes themselves.

Child Abuse Reporting Laws

In most circumstances, the principle of confidentiality keeps a patient's report to a therapist of criminal behavior from being reported by the therapist (7). However, the requirement to report child abuse supersedes the expectation of confidentiality in each of the 55 jurisdictions in the United States, District of Columbia, and territories. Although laws requiring that child abuse be reported have many important provisions and principles in common, they also have some important differences. Exploring all these laws in detail is beyond the scope of this chapter. However, a summary review of the differences among the states on key points in the laws is instructive.

Table 2 lists the key elements of child abuse reporting laws and shows where there are similarities and differences (8). It highlights differences in who is required to report, what one is required to report, what happens as a result of the report, and what happens to the reporter for reporting or for failing to report. A few of the points in this table are worthy of special note, to illustrate the complexities involved in understanding what is required and what the reporting process involves.

Defining Mandated Reporters

Some states qualify definitions of mandated reporters by stating that reporters must have learned of the reportable condition in the course of their "ordinary professional activities." In these states, a physician who overhears a neighbor abusing a child is not required to report, since the physician did not learn of the abuse in the practice of medicine. Wisconsin requires that the professional actually have seen the child professionally (9). Other states do not make this exception.

Defining Abuse

States vary tremendously in the details of their definitions of reportable conditions. Some states delineate long lists of specific findings that indicate abuse or neglect, whereas others do not define abuse and neglect at all. Most are somewhere in the middle. Statutes vary in how they address the issues of "threatened harm," emo-

Table 2. Key elements of child abuse reporting laws

Feature of law	Specific provision	No. of jurisdictions
Who must report	Any person knowing of abuse or neglect:	26
	Physicians	55
	Social workers	55
	Nurses	55
	Psychologists	47
	Other therapists	36
What must be reported	Physical abuse	55
	Sexual abuse	55
	Emotional injury	49
	Neglect	55
	Must be perpetrated by parent or other responsible person	36
	Defined only by child's state, any perpetrator is reportable	19
	Perpetrator's identity reported	40
	Reporter's identity reported	15
To whom must report be made	Child protective service (CPS) or social service	30
	Law enforcement	9
	Either social service or law enforcement, depending on nature of problem	
	or preference of reporter	25

Consequences of report	
If report made to law enforcement, it notifies CPS	18
If report made to CPS, it notifies law enforcement:	
In all cases	24
For sexual abuse	10
For fatalities	25
In emergency	2
On request of law enforcement	5
In various other specified situations	21
Child can be taken into immediate protective custody:	
By law enforcement	51
By CPS	32
By M.D. or hospital	26
By other court appointee	17
Penalties	
Failure to report is a misdemeanor punishable by fine and/or jail	51
Explicit establishment of civil liability for damages after failure to report	7
Implicit civil liability possible	55

Source. From Clearinghouse on Child Abuse and Neglect Information: State child abuse and neglect laws: a comparative analysis 1985. Washington, DC, U.S. Department of Health and Human Services, National Center for Child Abuse and Neglect, 1987.

tional abuse or "mental injury," and the problem of abuse occurring in the past.

Among the states that define abuse and neglect at all, about half indicate that the reportable condition is not only a current state of being harmed, but also the condition of being at risk for harm. Most states simply include this "at risk" condition by defining child abuse as "harm or threatened harm" stemming from a variety of specific acts or failures by parents or other caregivers. A few states define more specific conditions of risk in greater detail. The Wyoming reporting statute (10), for example, states that

> "abuse" means . . . harm or imminent danger to . . . a child . . . or substantial risk thereof; . . . "substantial risk" means a strong possibility as contrasted with a remote or insignificant possibility; "imminent danger" includes threatened harm and means a statement, overt act, condition or status which represents an immediate and substantial risk of sexual abuse or physical or mental injury. (p. 803)

In states in which risk or threat of harm is not part of the definition of what must be reported, it appears that the threshold for reporting is intended to be that abuse has already occurred. It usually also includes a requirement that some harm has occurred as a result of the abuse. In these states, reporting may be seen as a device appropriate for preventing further harm, but not as a way to prevent abuse from occurring at all. It is not clear whether leaving risk status out of the definitions of reportable conditions is intended to reflect an orientation away from prevention of abuse or is simply a practical way of keeping the threshold for reporting from being so low as to encourage spurious reporting of situations that are only potentially risky.

Case Example 1

A 9-year-old boy was referred to a psychiatrist for evaluation because of multiple behavior problems. Evaluation consisted of interviews with him, his 12-year-old brother, and his mother. Both the patient and his brother explicitly reported that they were generally unsupervised by their mother. His brother reported that the boy was frequently involved in risky activities with older, more antisocial neighborhood youths and had on several occasions been beaten up as a result. The boys' mother was seriously depressed and irritable and also appeared cognitively impaired. She reported that she had been involved with a protective service agency but seemed to be getting little help from them. She expressed extreme frustration with the boy, acknowledged that she used physical punishment with him, and said that at times she was so furious with him that she tried to hit him as hard as she could with no regard for consequences.

The evaluator expressed his concerns for the children's well-being to the mother and asked for her consent (which was not legally required) that he contact the protective service agency. She gave it. He reported the case to the protective service agency on the basis of apparent physical abuse and the risk caused by the mother's depression, irritability, impulsiveness, and lack of supervision. In the protective service investigation, the mother denied being physically abusive. The report was unsubstantiated. No evidence of abuse was found, and the mother's minimal compliance with protective service argued against the presence of neglect. The family failed to keep further appointments. In a follow-up telephone call, the mother expressed anger and dismay at having been reported, despite having consented to the report.

In this jurisdiction, risk or threatened harm is not a cause for action. Only actual harm resulting from abuse or neglect is a basis for intervention.

Almost all jurisdictions include mental or emotional harm resulting from abuse as a reportable condition. Two issues are ambiguous here. The first is whether including "emotional harm resulting from abuse" means that emotional *abuse* is explicitly reportable, or whether it means that the negative emotional *consequences* of physical or sexual abuse are reportable conditions. Some states explicitly define emotional or psychological abuse as reportable. Missouri, for example, defines abuse as

> any physical injury, sexual abuse, or emotional abuse inflicted on a child other than by accidental means by those responsible for his care, custody, and control. . . . (11, p. 440)

In contrast, Massachusetts's definition of the reportable condition is that a professional has

> reasonable cause to believe that a child . . . is suffering serious physical or emotional injury resulting from abuse inflicted upon him including sexual abuse, or from neglect, including malnutrition, or who is determined to be physically dependent upon an addictive drug at birth. . . . (12, p. 384)

This definition might be interpreted as indicating that emotional abuse per se is not a reportable condition, but rather that emotional *injury*, stemming from forms of abuse that are not further defined, is.

The second source of ambiguity regarding definitions of emotional abuse is that some statutes that attempt greater specificity seem to imply that the mere presence of emotional disturbance indicates emotional abuse and is reportable. For example, the Maine statute defines abuse as

> a threat to a child's health . . . by physical, mental or emotional injury or impairment . . . as evidenced by serious harm; . . . "serious harm" means . . . serious mental or emotional injury or *impairment* [emphasis added] which now or in the future is likely to be evidenced by serious mental, behavioral or personality disorder, including severe anxiety, depression or withdrawal, untoward aggressive behavior, seriously delayed development or similar serious dysfunctional behavior. . . . (13, p. 352)

This very detailed account of conditions of emotional impairment seems to have become disconnected from an abusive cause. It appears to indicate that virtually any child psychiatry patient in Maine is a reportable case of abuse.

Whether abuse that occurred in the past and is not ongoing must be reported is not addressed explicitly by any of the 55 statutes. A few laws define reportable abuse in the present tense, suggesting that past abuse need not be reported. More define reportable abuse as something that has occurred, suggesting that at least some events in the past must be reported. Others define the reportable condition as injury rather than abuse itself, such as the Massachusetts law quoted above. This definition could be interpreted to mean that the abuse could have happened at any time in the child's life and always continues to be reportable as long as the child continues to suffer from its effects (9,14,15).

Case Example 2

A seriously dysfunctional alcoholic and mentally ill man entered treatment as a result of a court case alleging that his two sons were in need of care and protection. Allegations focused on his wife's physical abuse of the children. He continued in treatment for years, through reunion of the family and dismissal of the case, with no further indications of physical abuse. His clinical condition, however, continued to be quite unstable. His marriage finally ended, and the court became reinvolved because of concerns about neglect of the children, who appeared to have substantial emotional problems. The patient became homeless and had virtually no contact with the boys, the older of whom entered a residential treatment center.

After being in the center for many months, the older boy reported that some years before his father had sexually abused him. The case treatment center reported the abuse to protective services, and the report of abuse was substantiated.

In this case, the abuse was years in the past and there was no current risk to the child from the father. Nor was there any risk to any other identifiable victims. There was, therefore, no clear protective issue in making this report. However, because it was determined that there had been abuse, and presumably that the boy was hurt by it, the report was substantiated.

Recent change in Maryland law exempts therapists of pedophiles from the requirement to report past sexual abuse that they have learned of from their patient, but only if the abuse occurred before the time that treatment began (16). Any abuse the patient reports occurring after the start of treatment must still be reported, even if it occurred significantly before it is reported.

Even in jurisdictions that define the reporting requirement in terms of present harm or risk, past abuse may be subject to report.

Case Example 3

In a case heard by the Montana Supreme Court (17), a group therapy patient acknowledged in a group session that her husband had sexually abused their daughters 16 years previously. Although by this time all the children were adults, the therapist reported the case as a mandatory child abuse report. The patient sued the therapist for violating her confidentiality by reporting, as the abuse was in the distant past. The therapist maintained that she was concerned for the possible risk to the patient's grandchildren.

The law requires reports when reporters "have reasonable cause to suspect that a child known to them in their professional . . . capacity is an abused . . . child" (18). Though this appears to be a fairly restrictive threshold for reporting, the court found that, in this situation, the therapist's report on behalf of potential current victims was appropriate.

An interesting sideline of the problems of defining abuse is the role of corporal punishment. Most statutes do not address the issue directly. Some make explicit that injuries occurring from excessive corporal punishment are reportable, suggesting that those occurring from nonexcessive corporal punishment may not be. South Carolina law addresses this problem in exceptional detail. Abuse includes

> injuries sustained as a result of excessive corporal punishment, but excluding corporal punishment or physical discipline which meets each of the following guidelines: (a) The physical aggression must be administered by a parent or person in loco parentis. (b) It must be perpetrated for the sole purpose of restraining or correcting the child. (c) The force or violence of the discipline must be reasonable in manner and moderate in degree. (d) The force and violence of the discipline must not have brought about permanent or lasting damage to the child. (e) The behavior of the parent must not be reckless or grossly negligent. (19, p. 653)

These detailed guidelines for acceptable physical punishment are a rare articulation of a local standard of acceptable practice in an area that in most statutes is vague and problematic.

The other area of interest in defining abuse is the role of the perpetrator. In many states, only abuse committed by parents or other responsible caregivers is reportable. Abuse committed by strangers or by older children is not covered by the reporting law and must be dealt with in other ways.

To Whom Must Report Be Made

States vary considerably in how they manage the reporting and investigative process. Some have all reports made either to protective services or to law enforcement; others leave this decision to the reporter. In many states, different conditions call for reports to different agencies, and reports to different agencies have different consequences. Involvement of law enforcement may increase the likelihood that an abuser will face prosecution. Even without prosecution, however, it may affect the abuser's response to the reporting experience and his or her likelihood of accepting the report as helpful. As indicated in the "consequences of report" section of Table 2, the initial destination of the report does not necessarily determine the limits of its availability. In most states, an initial report to protective services will be forwarded to law enforcement in at least some circumstances.

Case Example 2 (continued)

After the protective service agency substantiated the report of past sexual abuse in the case example 2 described earlier, the agency transmitted the information to the district attorney for consideration for prosecution, as the statute requires. When the patient learned of the allegations, he was shocked and maintained that nothing like what his son described had ever happened. When he learned that the police were after him, he became more acutely paranoid and fled the state.

In this case, the only outcome of the child abuse report was to generate criminal prosecution. This was not successful in clarifying the facts of the case, healing wounds in the family, or supporting treatment for the father. The father's treatment ended when he fled to avoid prosecution.

Penalties

Only Maryland, Mississippi, North Carolina, and Wyoming do not make failure to report abuse a misdemeanor. Potential penalties are small fines or short jail terms, but these are rarely invoked (20–22).

Case Example 4

A case receiving some notoriety in Massachusetts involved sexual abuse of several adolescent boys by a teacher in an exclusive private school (23). This case is the first and reportedly the only case in Massachusetts in which a mandated reporter has been prosecuted for failing to report child abuse (24).

According to newspaper reports, a male teacher who had taught in the same private school for 22 years was discovered to have involved some of his early-adolescent male students in masturbatory activities, and at least one other boy (his nephew, who was not a student at the school) in an extended relationship involving sexual activity. When the school headmaster learned of these activities, he fired the teacher but did not inform protective services. Reportedly, he was concerned for the privacy of the students involved and had concluded that the reporting threshold—that children were "suffering serious physical or emotional injury"—had not been met. The mother of the teacher's nephew notified protective services, but accounts are not clear as to whether this report was substantiated. She later contacted the district attorney, and a full investigation was undertaken, which led to prosecution of the teacher for rape, to which he ultimately pleaded guilty. The headmaster also admitted to sufficient facts and paid a $1,000 fine for not having made the required report.

Part of the school's justification for not having originally made the report appears to have been that the teacher's nephew was not a student at the school. Although the headmaster knew of the nephew's victimization, and that his emotional injury appeared to be more serious than that of the students, he did not report, apparently because his knowledge had not come in the course of his ordinary professional activities, i.e., it did not involve a student. Indeed, the school policy articulated by a task force after the legal action averred

that in the future "if there is reasonable cause to believe that if a
student at the school *[emphasis added] under the age of eighteen
is suffering serious physical or emotional injury resulting from abuse"
it would be reported.*

*If the headmaster had chosen to contest the prosecution for
failing to report, the limit set on the obligation to report by the
"ordinary professional activity" phrase might have been clarified.
This issue remains somewhat unclear, since the decision not to contest the charge does not necessarily mean the school was wrong in
its interpretation.*

Greater potential monetary consequences stem from a therapist's potential civil liability for damages occurring to a child as
a result of abuse that should have been reported and was not (3,
25). Such liability is explicitly established only in the statutes of
Arkansas, Iowa, Michigan, Montana, New York, and Rhode Is-
land. However, a California Supreme Court case in 1976, *Landeros
v. Flood* (26), established a precedent of negligence liability for
failure to report even in states that do not establish this liability
by statute, on the principle that among the duties owed to a patient
is the duty to report recognized child abuse. Some see this as an
expanding area of litigation in coming years, as a result of the
general increase in awareness of child abuse and its damaging consequences (27,28). However, this growth has not yet developed.

Case Example 5

Landeros v. Flood *is the best-known case of civil tort liability
related to failure to report child abuse. In this major decision, the
California Supreme Court made two important rulings. It established that damages stemming from failure to diagnose child abuse
could be the basis for a malpractice action. Perhaps more importantly, it established that a mandatory reporter who recognizes
abuse and fails to report it can be found to have been negligent for
failure to report, and therefore liable for damages resulting from
the abuse.*

*In this case, a child was seen in an emergency room with injuries
suggesting abuse, but a full exploration for signs of abuse was not
conducted and the diagnosis was not made. The child returned*

home, was further injured, seen in another hospital, diagnosed as abused, reported to protective services, and placed away from her mother who was ultimately convicted of child abuse.

The court found that the physician could be sued for negligence in failing to make the diagnosis and could also be sued for negligence in not making the required report if he had made the diagnosis. It determined that a requirement for a finding of negligence in not reporting per se (and by implication for a finding of guilt if there were a criminal charge for nonreporting) was that the doctor rec-ognized the abuse. He could not be held accountable for failing to report if he did not recognize the abuse, though he could be held liable for failing to recognize it.

All statutes provide immunity from civil suit for breach of confidentiality against mental health professionals who make re-quired reports. A few suits against other personnel for poor prac-tices in dealing with child abuse allegations have reached the courts (29,30). However, as long as reports have been made in good faith and with care (31), courts have consistently upheld immunity for mandated reporters (21).

This selected review of the child abuse reporting requirements in various states indicates that significant differences exist among them. Some of these individual features may be important when deciding whether reporting is required in a situation of potential violence or harm involving a child. Other features will be relevant to the question of whether reporting may be expected to succeed in protecting a child. No one can expect to be able to have a clear understanding of required reporting, or of what one can expect after reporting, without knowing both the laws in his or her own state and the usual practices of protective service and law enforce-ment agencies.

Issues in Therapist Responses

With this exploration of the variations in child abuse reporting requirements and consequences, and of the potential for civil lia-bility for damages occurring to patients or perpetrated by them, we can return to the basic typology of potential violence situations and look in more detail at the practical and ethical issues involved in them.

In situations involving child perpetrators, the therapist has some obligation to help protect potential victims. The obligation to protect is less distant when the victim is the adult patient of the therapist, but the therapist's actions are constrained somewhat in this situation by the desires of the patient. If the perpetrator is the patient's own child, the patient is likely to be particularly ambivalent about taking aggressive legal action against the child, even to protect himself or herself.

Under these conditions, the therapist owes no duty of confidentiality to the child. The therapist does owe the patient confidentiality, and unless the patient agrees to it, this duty will interfere with the therapist's conveying information to authorities that might help to get the child under control. The therapist should explore clinically with the patient his or her concerns about taking action against the child and help the patient evaluate the reasonableness of these concerns. For example, a parent may be concerned that bringing an action against a child for assault will result in the child's going to jail, suffering abuse, and receiving no help. If the therapist knows whether this outcome is likely, he or she can help the patient to decide; if the therapist does not know, it may be helpful to encourage the parent to seek legal consultation. If the parent's concern is that he or she will be overwhelmed by anxiety and guilt in pursuing action against the child, the therapist may help by exploring the roots of this anxiety and by helping him or her to evaluate the true likelihood that taking action would ultimately be helpful to the child.

Case Example 6

A mother was seen in the context of evaluating her school-age child for behavior problems. The mother reported that her older adolescent child, who was not seen, had been mentally ill. That child was currently at home without treatment, behaving in a menacing manner toward the mother.

Although the context of the evaluation was a juvenile court clinic, the juvenile court did not have jurisdiction over issues involving the older mentally ill adolescent. As a result, there was no direct action the psychiatrist could take to protect the mother (and other family members) through the younger child's court involvement. Instead, the psychiatrist encouraged the mother to seek help from the local court with appropriate jurisdiction in the form of a restraining order in a domestic violence action or an order to have the son examined for the purpose of civil mental health commitment.

In this situation, the patient (the mother) was pleased to follow the advice and to allow the evaluator to communicate his impressions of her situation and likely need for protection to representatives of the other court and of the mental health center involved in providing commitment and care for the son.

Two special circumstances deserve attention in the situation of a child threatening an adult patient. The first is that the therapist may have an obligation to go beyond the ordinary therapeutic relationship to act to protect the adult victim, if the victimization is serious and if the patient is impaired from self-protection by virtue of mental illness. Under such circumstances, the patient might be seen as representing a risk to himself or herself and require civil commitment for protection from (and treatment for) the consequences of his or her mental illness. The second is that, in many situations where a child is posing a threat to an adult, the child may have been or may still be suffering from abuse or neglect. In such situations, the therapist has an obligation to report and may have an obligation in every case to make a reasonable effort to determine if abuse or neglect of the child is an issue.

When the child patient is putting others at risk, the obligation to protect is not to the patient, but to third parties, according to the *Tarasoff* principle. Sometimes the therapist can meet this obligation effectively without breaking confidentiality with the patient. In other situations, clinical action within the therapeutic relationship will not be sufficient to protect others and the therapist will need to take actions that involve others with the child, such as warnings, commitment, or involving police and courts. In taking such actions, the therapist should have in mind the basic principle that it will almost always be in the patient's interest to be prevented from harming other people. Further, in some circumstances, the actions the therapist may take to protect others may be the same actions that will be of clinical benefit to the patient's treatment. In many circumstances, these would include hospitalizing the patient. In some circumstances, these would include involving police and courts in a manner that would enable the patient to be committed through the juvenile or criminal justice systems to nonhospital programs to provide both containment and appropriate socializing treatment. Before taking such action, the therapist should be informed as to the likelihood of such a therapeutic placement outcome, so that he or she can balance accurately the questions of the child's own long-range developmental interests and those of community protection.

Case Example 7

A 12-year-old boy was referred for psychopharmacological consultation by his therapist in a local child mental health agency. His mother originally brought him for treatment because of her concerns that he was involving younger children in the neighborhood in sexual activity. His therapist had been working with him on an outpatient basis without great success and was concerned about his depression. His mother recognized that the boy was both disturbed and potentially destructive to the younger children, but her most acute concern was that her son was at risk in the community of being beaten or killed by relatives of his younger child victims.

Although it did seem that antidepressant medication might be a useful part of the boy's treatment, it also appeared that the acute need was to protect both the boy and his victims from his sexual abuse and their potential reprisals. The protective service agency was already involved in the case, and the consultant and therapist worked together with the agency to place the boy in a therapeutic residential school with other children his own age. Though it was thought that he would be at somewhat less risk of sexually abusing peers in the program, an important consideration in making this placement was warning the residential program of his problem and thus of his need for special supervision to protect other residents.

As noted above, if the child's victim is also a child, the therapist may have a child abuse reporting obligation as well. A detailed review of reporting statutes indicates that this obligation will only exist in jurisdictions that do not limit the reporting requirement to situations involving abuse by a parent or other responsible adult. However, even if reporting is not required by the statute, the therapist should consider whether reporting would likely serve to protect the victim. If it would, then it is a reasonable course to pursue. In most circumstances, the therapist would be immune from litigation regarding breach of confidentiality and would also discharge the *Tarasoff* obligation. If a report of actual or potential child abuse will be unlikely to provide real protection and could be expected to disrupt the patient's treatment, then the only reason to make such a report would be if a local statute required it (and the therapist preferred compliance with the law to informal civil disobedience) (32,33).

Whatever action a child's therapist may take to protect a child's potential victim, the therapist should routinely consider involving the child's parent in the action (34). This involvement should include at least informing the parent of the risk posed by the child and of the therapist's actions to reduce it. Ideally, it would include actions the parent would take to reduce the risk as well. This involvement may break the patient's confidentiality, but it would do so in a manner that is certainly acceptable, given the parent's legitimate interest in the child's condition and progress. The therapist should *not* involve the parent only if the therapist has firm ground for believing that informing the parent would reduce the chances of being able to offer successful protection. In any such situation, the therapist should carefully consider whether the belief that parent involvement would not help indicates that the child is suffering from parental neglect.

Situations involving children at risk of being harmed create more complex problems, again involving the differences between duties to patients and duties to potential victims, as well as a thorough understanding of the processes in reporting child abuse.

When a child patient appears at risk of being harmed, the therapist may have an explicit duty to the state to report on the basis of child abuse (depending on the specific statute). He or she also has duties to the patient, including maintaining the patient's confidentiality and providing appropriate professional help to reduce the risk to the patient.

Case Example 8

An 11-year-old boy was brought for evaluation by his mother because of school problems and a bad attitude at home. She was very frustrated and angry with him. She had gone out of her way to try to understand him and nothing seemed to work. The school repeatedly called her in to report her son's problems. She described using physical punishment with him, since nothing else seemed to work, and she acknowledged sometimes being quite severe. She was otherwise attentive, thoughtful, and supportive of her son's appropriate development and socialization.

The boy was unusually intelligent, and it soon became clear that part of his problem was that he was bored in school and making school personnel angry by demanding attention. He complained with some bitterness about his mother's beatings and about her criticism of him, but also showed warmth and pleasure in relating with her. There was no indication that he was suffering serious physical injury as a result of being beaten.

The mother reported a previous attempt at treatment that she had found marginally useful but had stopped in response to the therapist making a child abuse report. The report had been investigated and not substantiated, but she had felt hurt, misunderstood, and unsupported both by the therapist's report and by the protective service investigation.

In the current encounter, the clinician considered making a report of child abuse. She determined, however, that the threshold of serious injury was not clearly met. She felt that it was reasonable to expect that appropriate clinical and educational services would provide whatever protection of the child's interests was truly needed, and that making a report was much more likely to be harmful than helpful to the child. She contracted with the family for a simple behavior management intervention, which quickly succeeded in reducing conflict and physical punishment in the family. She worked with the family and school system to arrange a more appropriately challenging individualized school program. Within several months, both mother and son were substantially more comfortable and successful in dealing with one another and there were no longer questions of abuse.

The duty to protect the patient may be discharged by making

a child abuse report, if it is reasonable to believe that such a report will help reduce the risk. However, in discharging the obligation to the patient, the therapist must responsibly assess whether reporting will actually help, or whether it may make the situation even worse.

Reporting itself can be harmful in several ways. Because in reporting the therapist necessarily fails in his obligation to maintain the patient's confidentiality, reporting may undermine the child's or family's confidence and trust in the therapist, interfering with the potential benefit of treatment. It may threaten the autonomy of the relationship between child and parent, especially by leading to removal of the child from the parent's care and placement in state care, with some attendant risk for exposure to other kinds of neglect and abuse. It may even lead to criminal prosecution of the parent, with the child as prosecuting witness responsible for the parent's incarceration (35). It may in these ways lead to further victimization of the child and create serious interference with the child's own development of a sense of mastery of difficult situations.

These problems create difficulty for the therapist's alliance with the child. In addressing this difficulty, the therapist should attend to the child's understanding of the situation and to the child's feelings about the reporting process and about what may ensue. The therapist should also determine what should be the appropriate level of credit to give to the child's desires and judgment in dealing with these problems. Some children will resist outside involvement and the possibility of placement out of generalized anxiety or pathological attachment to an abusing parent; others may foster accusations against parents in a poorly socialized manipulative attempt to gain freedom from appropriate limits. In either case, the therapist's decision to report and involve outside agencies may go against the desires of the child and may thus interfere with the child's comfort in the therapeutic relationship. Ideally, the struggle with the therapist over reporting can foster the child's growth, but in many cases it may just disrupt the therapy.

On the other hand, reporting may in some cases be the key to both providing immediate protection and fostering a stronger therapeutic alliance (36–38). The child may feel validated in concerns for his or her own health and safety and empowered to resist accepting abuse. Both child and parent may be relieved that the abuse has come to light and may as a result be more comfortable establishing a more complete and focused treatment contract. The reporting process may itself provide the occasion for the provision of additional services through a protective service agency. These services might otherwise have been unavailable to the child, either because of a parent's resistance or because the family was not entitled to services without protective issues having been identified.

When an adult patient is the perpetrator, the therapist faces the greatest apparent conflict of obligations. The obligation to maintain confidentiality is in direct conflict with the obligation the therapist may owe to the state to report child abuse (39). The obligation to third parties to protect them from potential harm by the patient exists regardless of whether the therapist must report the situation as child abuse. This duty to protect others may also interfere with confidentiality, though not always. Finally, there is a therapeutic obligation to the patient to consider the potential negative consequences for the patient of his or her doing harm to another. As part of the treatment alliance, the therapist should thus feel obliged to attend to and act to prevent harm on the patient's behalf.

Just as in the situation in which the child is the patient, the adult patient may have many possible reactions to a therapist's acting to protect others or reporting abuse to the state. These may range from paranoid outrage, termination of therapy, and major deterioration in functioning, to relief and gratitude to the therapist for taking the initiative to protect both the child and the patient. Obviously, the therapist will be better able to balance the potential conflicting interests involved in breaking confidentiality if he or she is able to make some assessment of the patient's likely response.

Case Example 9

A woman with a 3-year-old child was involved in court in a care and protection action on the child's behalf. She was referred for urgent consultation because she was extremely agitated. She acknowledged having discontinued her psychiatric medication. The court made it clear to her that although she had a right to refuse medication, her condition was such that the court would remove physical custody of the child unless she resumed medication and appropriate psychiatric treatment. She complied and began regular treatment meetings with a psychiatrist. She regained adequate control rapidly and did not lose physical custody of her child.

She continued in treatment for many months, complaining bitterly about taking medication that she did not want. Without informing the psychiatrist, she discontinued the medication, but did not show any deterioration in her condition for about 3 months. By the time she began to appear hypomanic again and acknowledged having stopped medication, she was pregnant, and medication was not recommended as long as she was in relative control. When she became acutely manic, she was hospitalized, where she continued to refuse medication. Her son remained at home in the husband's custody.

When she was discharged from the hospital she remained somewhat unstable, and there were questions as to whether she would return to her marriage. Though she remained involved with the court and with protective services, her treatment had been confidential. At this point it was clear that more active monitoring involvement by the protective service agency would be necessary to ensure that her condition did not put her son at substantial risk when she returned home. After discussing these concerns with her, the therapist contacted the protective service agency and established a plan with the agency, the court, and the therapist for monitoring her condition. This plan required the therapist to keep the agency and the court informed regarding her condition.

This was not a situation in which the therapist risked disrupting therapy by introducing the notion of reporting child abuse for the first time. The patient was familiar with the process and had established a relationship with the therapist. She felt him to be helpful to her in meeting the requirements of the court so that she could retain custody of her child. In the current situation, she was not at all dismayed at the prospect of having her privacy disrupted, because she was familiar with the other actors involved and understood quite well the benefits to herself in cooperating with the agency and the court.

Unlike the situation of the child patient at risk, the formal protecting duties in this situation are not to the patient, but rather to potential victims. Therefore, the therapist's attention to the patient's own desires regarding reporting or other actions taken to protect a potential child victim is different. In the child patient situation, the concern for the patient's desires rests on the principle that actions taken to protect are taken in the patient's interest as part of the therapist's treatment obligation to the patient. If the patient reasonably and competently does not want the therapist's help in this specific manner, the therapist should attend to this desire as part of contracting for treatment with the patient. With an adult perpetrator patient, the protective actions are not primarily taken for the patient's benefit, but rather for the victim's. Therefore, a patient's objection to taking protective action should not be given the credit it might deserve if the patient were the victim. The therapist ought to attend to the patient's objections as feelings, and even as potential indicators of the patient's likely response to the therapist's action. However, the therapist should not act or fail to act on the basis of the patient's objections, because the duty at issue is not a duty to further the interests of the patient.

Because of conflicts between a therapist's duty to maintain confidentiality and other duties, a therapist may have to break confidentiality. Therefore, some observers have suggested that, in the process of contracting for treatment, the therapist should clearly inform the patient as to the limits of confidentiality and under what circumstances it could be broken (15,20,40). A recent change in the licensing law for psychologists in Massachusetts (41) requires that psychologists give this information to all patients at the beginning of any professional consultation. Surveys of therapists' practices in these areas have found that many therapists are not very familiar with reporting requirements and may not be able to anticipate their own actions if issues of risk emerge in treatment (42,43). As a result, they may actually be unable to let patients know what to expect in a reliable way at the beginning of treatment.

Conclusions

Four principles are at issue in understanding therapists' obligations in dealing with potentially dangerous situations involving children and families. Therapists must strive to maintain the patient's confidentiality. They have a duty to protect third parties from identifiable and predictable dangers posed by the patient. They have a somewhat more ambiguous duty to take action to protect the patient from certain identifiable threats posed by others, as a part of the general duty to provide care and treatment. Finally, they are obliged, under conditions that vary by location, to report child abuse.

Reviewing these principles in situations involving therapy of children and families indicates that they tend to put conflicting pressures on therapists. Simple or general advice is not adequate for resolving these conflicts, since each case is different clinically and presents different potential problems and opportunities. None of the principles is unambiguous, and no specific actions are recommended as guaranteed to either work or be correct. Sometimes maintaining confidentiality is of utmost importance. Sometimes everyone's interests are best served by breaking it. It is naive to think that reporting child abuse will always succeed in protecting a child or in strengthening the therapist's alliance with the "healthy" parts of a child or parent. It is equally naive to imagine that reporting or otherwise breaking confidentiality to provide protection will always have a disruptive and damaging effect on treatment. It is both naive and professionally arrogant to assume that a break of confidentiality that disrupts treatment will not be outweighed by other benefits. Protection or other services might be more valuable to a child or family than confidential treatment. It is equally naive to imagine that breaking confidentiality will always succeed in providing a family with these benefits (21).

No adequate empirical research is available to tell us with certainty for which children and families it will be most important to maintain confidentiality, either for effective treatment or for protection, and for which it will be more effective to break it. It is difficult to conceive ethical ways to conduct experiments that might actually provide this information. As a result, therapists must use their clinical judgment as best they can, taking care to consider the wide range of clinical and ethical variables involved. It is hoped that readers will not be demoralized by the problems in resolving these principles, but instead will be challenged to examine them seriously case by case and, as a result, be able to respond to the needs of children and families with greater sensitivity and effectiveness.

References

1. Smith SR, Meyer RG: Child abuse reporting laws and psychotherapy: a time for reconsideration. Int J Law Psychiatry 7:351–366, 1984
2. Bernstein AH: Child abuse reports: breach of medical confidentiality? Hospitals 58:86–88, 1984
3. Schroeder LO: Legal liability: a professional concern. Clinical Social Work Journal 7:194–199, 1979
4. Beck JC: When the patient threatens violence: an empirical study of clinical practice after *Tarasoff*. Bull Am Acad Psychiatry Law 10:189–201, 1982
5. Appelbaum PS: *Tarasoff* and the clinician: problems in fulfilling the duty to protect. Am J Psychiatry 142:425–429, 1985
6. Carlson RJ, Friedman LC, Riggert SC: The duty to warn/protect: issues in clinical practice. Bull Am Acad Psychiatry Law 15:179–186, 1987
7. Appelbaum PS, Meisel A: Therapists' obligations to report their patients' criminal acts. Bull Am Acad Psychiatry Law 14:221–230, 1986
8. Clearinghouse on Child Abuse and Neglect Information: State child abuse and neglect laws: a comparative analysis 1985. Washington, DC, U.S. Department of Health and Human Services, National Center for Child Abuse and Neglect, 1987
9. Miller RD, Weinstock R: Conflict of interest between therapist-patient confidentiality and the duty to report sexual abuse of children. Behavioral Sciences and the Law 5:161–174, 1987
10. Wyoming Statutes Annotated § 14-3-202(a)(ii); cited in Missouri Revised Statutes 5.210.110(1) (1986); cited in Clearinghouse on Child Abuse and Neglect Information: State statutes 1986: definitions of abuse and neglect: reporting laws. Washington, DC, U.S. Department of Health and Human Services, National Center for Child Abuse and Neglect, 1987, p 803
11. Missouri Revised Statutes 5.210.110(1) (1986); cited in Clearinghouse on Child Abuse and Neglect Information: State statutes 1986: definitions of abuse and neglect: reporting laws. Washington, DC, U.S. Department of Health and Human Services, National Center for Child Abuse and Neglect, 1987, p 440

12. Massachusetts General Laws Chapter 119 § 51A; cited in Clearinghouse on Child Abuse and Neglect Information: State statutes 1986: definitions of abuse and neglect: reporting laws. Washington, DC, U.S. Department of Health and Human Services, National Center for Child Abuse and Neglect, 1987, p 384
13. Maine Revised Statutes Annotated title 22, § 4002(10) (Supp 1986); cited in Clearinghouse on Child Abuse and Neglect Information: State statutes 1986: definitions of abuse and neglect: reporting laws. Washington, DC, U.S. Department of Health and Human Services, National Center for Child Abuse and Neglect, 1987, p 352
14. Weinstock R, Weinstock D: Child abuse reporting trends: an unprecedented threat to confidentiality. J Forensic Sci 33:418–431, 1988
15. Kelly RJ: Limited confidentiality and the pedophile. Hosp Community Psychiatry 38:1046–1048, 1987
16. Maryland Laws 1987 Chapter 635 § 2(b)
17. Gross v Myers, 748 P2d 459 (Mont 1987)
18. § 41-3-201(1) and (2) MCA (1985)
19. South Carolina Code Annotated 20–7–490(c)(1) (Supp 1986); cited in Clearinghouse on Child Abuse and Neglect Information: State statutes 1986: definitions of abuse and neglect: reporting laws. Washington, DC, U.S. Department of Health and Human Services, National Center for Child Abuse and Neglect, 1987, p 653
20. Butz RA: Reporting child abuse and confidentiality in counseling. Social Casework 66:83–90, 1985
21. Clearinghouse on Child Abuse and Neglect Information: Review of 1987 child abuse and neglect case law. Washington, DC, U.S. Department of Health and Human Services, National Center for Child Abuse and Neglect, 1988
22. Smith v State, No C85–1599 (Nev Dist Ct 1986)
23. Gagen T: School secret. Boston Globe Magazine, July 3, 1988, pp 14–29
24. Beck M, J.D.: Office of Massachusetts Attorney General, and Devine S, J.D., Office of General Counsel, Massachusetts Department of Social Services, personal communications, 1989
25. Guyer MJ: Child abuse and neglect statutes: legal and clinical implications. Am J Orthopsychiatry 52:73–81, 1982
26. Landeros v Flood, 551 P2d 389, 17 Cal3d 399 (Cal Supreme Ct 1976)
27. Benedek E: Emerging issues in forensic child psychiatry. Paper presented at Tufts-New England Medical Center Child Psychiatry Symposium, Boston, MA, November 9, 1984
28. Guyer M: New issues for litigation in forensic child psychiatry. Paper

presented at Midyear Institute, American Academy of Child and Adolescent Psychiatry, San Diego, CA, March 19, 1988

29. BeVier v Hucal, 806 F2d 123 (7th Cir 1986)
30. Turner v District of Columbia, No 85–634 (DC 1987)
31. Berkowitz S: Personal prejudices and legal liability. Massachusetts Psychological Association Newsletter, Oct 1988, p 6
32. Schoeman F, Reamer FG: Should child abuse always be reported? Hastings Cent Rep 13:19–20, 1983
33. Pope KS, Bajt TR: When laws and values conflict: a dilemma for psychologists. Am Psychol 43:828–829, 1988
34. Racusin RJ, Felsman JK: Reporting child abuse: the ethical obligation to inform parents. J Am Acad Child Psychiatry 25:485–489, 1986
35. Renshaw DC: Evaluating suspected cases of child sexual abuse. Psychiatric Annals 17:262–270, 1987
36. Green AH: Expanding psychiatry's role in child abuse treatment. Hosp Community Psychiatry 30:702–705, 1979
37. Wulsin LR, Bursztajn H, Gutheil TG: Unexpected clinical features of the *Tarasoff* decision: the therapeutic alliance and the duty to warn. Am J Psychiatry 140:601–603, 1983
38. Harper G, Irvin E: Alliance formation with parents: limit-setting and the effect of mandated reporting. Am J Orthopsychiatry 55:550–560, 1985
39. Brandon S: The psychiatrist in child abuse—ethical and role conflicts. Child Abuse Negl 3:401–405, 1979
40. Berlin FS: Laws on mandatory reporting of suspected child abuse (letter). Am J Psychiatry 145:1039, 1988
41. Massachusetts General Laws Chapter 112 § 129A
42. Swoboda JS, Elwork A, Sales BD, et al: Knowledge of and compliance with privileged communication and child-abuse reporting laws. Professional Psychology 9:448–457, 1978
43. Muehleman JT, Kimmons C: Psychologists' views on child abuse reporting, confidentiality, life, and the law: an exploratory study. Professional Psychology 12:631–638, 1981

CHAPTER SEVEN

Therapist Sexual Misconduct and the Duty to Protect

Spencer Eth, M.D.
Gregory B. Leong, M.D.

Sexual activity between psychotherapists and patients has attracted increasing attention (1,2) despite historic recognition that this behavior is inappropriate. Freud (3) noted that the rule of sexual abstinence during treatment is one in which "ethical motives unite with technical ones to restrain him [the psychoanalyst] from giving the patient his love" (p. 169). Several potentially serious psychological consequences have been identified after therapist-patient sexual contact, including worsening of interpersonal relationships, mistrust of the opposite sex and of therapists, sexual dysfunction, substance abuse, suicidality, and psychiatric hospitalization (4–6). The belief that psychotherapist-patient sexual contact is always or usually psychologically harmful to patients is shared by virtually all (97.4%) of the psychiatrists queried in a recent large survey of American Psychiatric Association (APA) members (7).

In this chapter, we consider whether the *Tarasoff* doctrine applies to situations in which a psychotherapist learns of the sexual misconduct of a colleague whose behavior places patients at risk for psychological harm from therapist-patient sexual contact. We will not address posttermination sexual relations, as ethical and legal status remain ambiguous in this situation. The application of the *Tarasoff* principle to professional misconduct may be viewed as a further step in the expansion of *Tarasoff* to areas seemingly far removed from the original case involving a psychotic patient posing a physical threat to an identifiable victim.

Briefly, *Tarasoff* refers to a cause of action for negligence against a psychotherapist for failing to protect an identifiable third party from the patient's violent attack (8). Several subsequent cases, popularly known as *Tarasoff*-type cases or *Tarasoff* progeny, have been adjudicated in other jurisdictions and have been extensively discussed elsewhere (9–11). Taken broadly, *Tarasoff*-type duty cases have allowed for the confidentiality of the psychotherapist-patient relationship to be breached where the overriding interest of the physical well-being of another person is at stake. Moreover, *Tarasoff* progeny have been extended to nonidentifiable third parties (12,13), property (14), and conceivably to the human immunodeficiency virus (HIV)–seropositive patient who persists in engaging in unsafe sexual practices (15). In fact, the APA has promulgated a similar stance in its AIDS confidentiality guidelines (16). Given this trend, the application of the *Tarasoff* model to alleged psychotherapist sexual misconduct is quite conceivable.

Psychotherapist-Patient Sexual Contact

The extent of the problem of therapist-patient contact has been estimated through surveys of psychologists and psychiatrists performed over the past 20 years. These surveys reflect similar rates and a nondeclining trend (1,2,17). In the most extensive survey of psychiatrists, Gartrell et al. (18) found that 7.1% of the 1,057 men and 3.1% of the 385 women questioned acknowledged sexual contact with their own patients, whereas Simon (19) believes the true prevalence could be as great as 15–25%. Gartrell et al. (18) found that one-third of the surveyed psychiatrists engaging in sexual activity with patients did so with more than one patient. This strongly suggests that the current patients of a therapist who has a history of sexual misconduct are at increased risk for sexual exploitation.

Consider the following case example:

Susan C is a 28-year-old single second-grade teacher who enters psychotherapy with Dr. A, a female psychiatrist, complaining of a series of masochistic relationships. She is frequently tearful in sessions as she describes her pattern of infatuation with inappropriate men.

Ms. C has had affairs with married men, older men, and occasionally with men from a lower social class. Ms. C usually convinces herself that her partner loves her and will treat her kindly, despite mounting evidence to the contrary. Inevitably, the affair ends with Ms. C feeling deceived, rejected, and worthless.

Ms. C traces her interpersonal difficulties to an unhappy childhood spent in the home of an erratic, alcoholic father. In the 4th month of treatment, she begins to share the details of her father's sexual advances. Starting when she was 7, Mr. C would visit his daughter's room weekly to "snuggle." She at first appreciated the affection, but later realized that "something was wrong" with the way she was being touched. When she was 9 years old, her father was killed in an automobile accident while intoxicated.

During a particularly intense session in the 9th month of therapy, Ms. C discloses her most closely guarded secret. Dr. A had known that Ms. C had been seen by a colleague for 6 months several years before. Ms. C finally was able to reveal that her former psychiatrist, Dr. B, had become intimate with her during treatment. In retrospect, she believes that the therapeutic relationship had become sexualized when Dr. B hugged her after an emotionally charged session. Before long they were embracing and stroking each other during the hour. Ms. C felt very special and important, and responded with sustained contentment to his many compliments. They had had sexual intercourse on five occasions when Ms. C noticed the announcement of Dr. B's wedding engagement in the local newspaper. Ms. C never returned to Dr. B's office.

Dr. A is impressed with her patient's sincerity and in the consistency of her repeated accounts of her sexual relationship with Dr. B. Although surprised by this material, Dr. A admits to herself that she can recall Dr. B's unsavory reputation for his seductive behavior toward women residents. Dr. B continues to practice in their community, presumably posing a risk to his female patients by his propensity for sexual indiscretion.

Although many patients who have been exploited by their therapists avoid further treatment, others, like Ms. C, do seek help, both for long-standing problems and specifically for symptoms arising from the sexual abuse. Thus, many psychotherapists could discover themselves in Dr. A's predicament. In fact, Gartrell et al. (20) reported that 65% of her total sample of 1,442 psychiatrists had treated at least one patient who had been sexually involved with a previous therapist. In 87% of these patients, the sexual contact had a harmful effect.

Although Dr. A's current patient is no longer endangered by her former psychiatrist, Dr. B's present patients remain at risk for psychological harm. What obligations does Dr. A have in this case, and how can they be reconciled with concerns about confidentiality? Not only is Dr. A's patient, Ms. C, entitled to confidentiality about her treatment, so are Dr. B's present patients. In practice, most psychiatrists in Dr. A's situation would take no direct action to protect Dr. B's current patients. Gartrell et al. (20) found that only 8% of all psychiatrists who knew of a colleague who engages in potentially harmful sexual misconduct reported him or her to a professional association or legal authority and only one, apparently, made an attempt to warn the patients at risk. Yet, these psychiatrists were in conflict over remaining passive, because 56% favored a policy of mandatory reporting of alleged sexual misconduct. Such a policy would compel the discovering psychiatrist to act. This position suggests a narrow view of the *Tarasoff* model by justifying mandatory reporting as the favored form of discharging the duty to protect despite an inherent conflict with the principle of confidentiality.

Analyzing the Tarasoff *Analogy*

There are noteworthy differences between sexual misconduct and the *Tarasoff* prototype. In the typical *Tarasoff* situation, there is a potential for physical harm. Psychotherapist-patient sex has virtually no potential for significant physical injury, even though the likelihood of psychological harm may be great. Further, the patient victim generally acquiesces to the sexual activity and, in some instances, is frankly seductive. This cooperative stance contrasts with the usual circumstances of rape in which the sexual act is perpetrated forcibly and without consent. Although some commentators, such as Masters and Johnson (21), contend that any therapist who seduces a patient, regardless of whether the seduction was initiated by patient or therapist, should be charged with rape, prosecution is rarely successful unless clear force or fear is used

(22). Only Minnesota and a few other states have criminalized psychotherapist-patient sexual contact (23).

It is important to distinguish two quite different clinical situations. One involves the patient who alleges sexual impropriety on the part of a former therapist. The second concerns whether a current patient poses a threat of foreseeable harm to a third party. In the latter instance, the patient–potential perpetrator is interviewed directly and under the auspices of the psychotherapist-patient relationship, whereas in the former there may be no opportunity to evaluate the alleged psychotherapist-perpetrator. In fact, the treating psychiatrist has only hearsay knowledge of the incident (24). The accusation may be a product of the patient's erotic fantasies or psychosis or may serve as a means of retaliating for perceived disappointment or rejection in the transference (25). In these cases, the patient poses a threat to the psychotherapist and not the reverse. If we are to afford our colleagues the usual judicial presumption of innocence, then establishing psychological dangerousness by the uncorroborated account of a patient would be problematic. Failing to demonstrate the threat with direct evidence would obviate any duty to protect hypothetical victims.

We do not find convincing arguments to support the application of the *Tarasoff* doctrine in these cases of sexual misconduct by a former therapist. If the court were to establish a duty to protect, how could a psychiatrist who learns of a colleague's sexual activity act to safeguard the other therapist's patients? In fact, the range of options available in this instance is much narrower than in the usual *Tarasoff* situation. Because the potentially dangerous psychiatrist, Dr. B, is not her patient, Dr. A cannot revise her treatment plan by adjusting medication dosage or by initiating steps to effect involuntary civil commitment (assuming such measures are even appropriate for patients whose threat of harm is psychological). Dr. A is powerless to exert behavior control over someone with whom she has no therapeutic relationship. Another limitation facing Dr. A is her inability to warn the persons at risk, even if she felt morally compelled to try. The identities of Dr. B's patients are known only to Dr. B and those individuals. Their anonymity cannot be pierced by the well-intentioned Dr. A or, perhaps, even by subpoena of their medical records.

The only viable recourse left open to Dr. A is to notify an

agency and request further action. Dr. A may choose to file an ethics complaint against Dr. B with the local district branch of the APA. This step presupposes that Dr. B is a member of the APA and subject to its review. Sexual contact with a patient constitutes a violation of Section 1 of the Principles of Medical Ethics With Annotations Especially Applicable to Psychiatry (26): "Sexual activity with a patient is unethical." The penalties for ethical misconduct range from admonishment to expulsion from the organization. A psychiatrist who becomes aware of unethical conduct by a colleague has an affirmative duty to "expose those physicians deficient in character or competence, or who engage in deception" (26). However, the psychiatrist is also bound by the rule requiring that doctor-patient confidentiality be honored "within the constraints of the law" (26).

It has been noted that impairment may reveal itself as sexual misconduct (27). Impaired therapists may be afflicted with depression, substance abuse, or family crises. From this perspective, a psychiatrist learning from a patient of a colleague's lapse of judgment might wish to personally confront the other therapist with the suspicion of impairment without revealing the source of information. By so doing, the psychiatrist has intervened to promote treatment of the "dangerous" colleague, thereby protecting the patients at risk. Consonant with this compassionate approach has been the establishment of medical society physician impairment committees and state licensing board–sanctioned diversion programs. Presently, California's diversion treatment program accommodates physicians suffering from substance abuse who may also be engaging in sexual relations with patients.

If Ms. C refuses to permit disclosure of her name, Dr. A may file an allegation of sexual misconduct against Dr. B but cannot identify the alleged victimized patient. The ethics committee of the district branch would be stymied. The accused psychiatrist may not know which of his patients is lodging the complaint, or if he did know or suspect who it was, he could not respond by providing clinical data without a consent from that patient or certainty about her identity. Thus, the ethics committee would be forced to operate without a patient personally complaining or a psychiatrist authorized to reply. In the absence of that evidence, the allegations would almost certainly have to be dropped. It is therefore critical that the patient file a detailed complaint containing a consent form that forces the accused psychiatrist to respond fully. One goal of the current treatment would be to resolve the conflicts that inhibit the patient from acting to redress the wrong he or she has suffered. If the patient does register a complaint, then that action frees the treating psychiatrist from the responsibility of acting in his or her place in a manner that would ultimately prove ineffective.

Dr. A could, in theory, also notify the police or state licensing board, although these authorities would also be handicapped in pursuing an investigation of an anonymous patient complaint. As mentioned earlier, the police are unlikely to consider consensual sexual activity between therapist and patient a criminal offense. A state licensing board, however, might treat such behavior as a serious matter, but only if given a sufficiently specific account of the sexual activity. That type of information should be provided by the patient-victim, relieving the psychiatrist in this instance of his or her *Tarasoff* responsibility.

A way of bypassing the need for the patient to file a formal complaint, and at the same time resolving the psychiatrist's ambivalence about acting, is through a mandatory reporting statute. Although a majority of psychiatrists surveyed endorsed mandatory reporting (20), only Minnesota has such a law in place (23). It requires the reporting of any physician who engages in sexual contact or seductive or demeaning behavior with a patient, while providing immunity for the physician-reporter. The sole exception is for information obtained from an offending physician during his or her treatment, if and only if that doctor has already limited the scope of his or her practice and no longer constitutes a threat. Mandatory reporting forces the psychiatrist to violate confidentiality regardless of the patient-victim's wishes. Vinson (28) described how a patient may feel "doubly used"—having been exploited first by a former therapist for sexual gratification and then by a subsequent therapist to satisfy a professional obligation. Similar mandatory reporting laws were enacted in response to the concerns about child abuse. They were generally designed to protect dependent children from future physical harm by a caregiver. Applying these inflexible laws to sexual misconduct sacrifices the competent adult patient's privacy interest in an unlikely effort to protect other competent adults from the risk of seduction by a therapist. Knowing that certain secrets cannot be kept may, in itself, deter sexually exploited patients from seeking treatment, while infantilizing those who expect to be afforded the consent rights of adults. Further, the problems attendant to false allegations as well as the inherent difficulties in adjudicating anonymous complaints all point to the severe limitations of mandatory reporting as a useful remedy.

As a sensible alternative to mandatory reporting, California has adopted a "brochure" statute (29,30). This code requires a psychotherapist whose patient alleges a history of sexual contact with a prior psychotherapist to provide and discuss a brochure that describes the definition of psychotherapist-patient sexual contact, common personal reactions and histories of victims and their families, patient's bill of rights, options and instructions for reporting the alleged sexual contact, complaint procedures available to the patient, and available support services. Failure to follow the California "brochure" law represents "unprofessional conduct."

The Offending Therapist in Treatment

By contrast to the situation in which sexual misconduct is reported by the former patient-victim, consider this case example:

Dr. Y is a middle-aged psychiatrist who decided to seek psychotherapy for a pervasive sense of boredom in his marriage and in his professional practice. Dr. Y had been in therapy once before, when his residency training director had recommended that he receive assistance for some prominent countertransference conflicts that were interfering with his treatment of severely disturbed patients. Dr. Y found at that time that therapy had restored his self-confidence and effectively placated his supervisors.

Dr. Y began to see Dr. X, a senior training analyst affiliated with the psychoanalytic institute in a nearby city. In one of his weekly sessions, Dr. Y revealed as an aside that he was having sexual relations with two of his current patients. Dr. X questioned Dr. Y's clinical judgment, but Dr. Y denied that the sexual contact was having any negative effects on his patients; in fact, he contended that it may be beneficial by relieving their symptoms of frigidity. Dr. Y's reaction to his therapist's criticism is consistent with Dr. X's diagnostic impression of a narcissistic personality. Dr. Y has frequently insisted that their sessions must be held in strictest confidence. Dr. X is especially troubled because Dr. Y's misconduct has to date gone unreported. Further, there is little likelihood that psychotherapy will have a remedial impact on Dr. Y's improper behavior.

This disclosure presents a grave challenge to Dr. X, who must certainly be aware of the danger Dr. Y poses to his patients. To our knowledge there is no record of litigation in precisely this area. Nonetheless, we anticipate that the psychiatrist who is informed directly about his or her patient's professional sexual misconduct and fails to respond could be held liable for damages in any subsequent negligence action. It is insufficient to merely continue the psychotherapy in the hope that treatment will eventually eradicate the sexual misconduct. If a physician-patient suffered from lapses of consciousness, the treating psychiatrist would have difficulty defending the decision not to report the loss of consciousness to the department of motor vehicles (31). Yet, according to Melella et al. (32), serious sex offenders, "perhaps more than any other group have the potential to harm victims" (p. 84). In these situations, the welfare of society can be seriously threatened. Hence, "confidentiality should and indeed must, be breached" (9).

In clinical practice, psychiatrists probably rarely act outside of treatment when managing therapist-patients who commit acts of sexual misconduct. Stone (33) described several cases of psychiatric residents who became romantically involved with their patients. *Tout comprendre, c'est tout pardonner* was offered as a reason why the hospital administration appeared reluctant to respond decisively. The behavior of these psychiatrists-in-training seemed understandable given their personality dynamics. What is explainable is all too often forgivable, and the offending therapist was usually spared. The proper action of a residency director may be to terminate the training. An appropriate response of a treating psychiatrist would be to report his or her patient-therapist to an ethics committee or state licensing board. It is, of course, impossible to warn an offending psychiatrist's patients, because their identities cannot be uncovered.

Our recommendation to the treating psychiatrist would result

in a breach of confidentiality that could have devastating consequences for the therapist-patient. Notifying a licensing board may
begin a process that leads to licensure revocation and the end of a
professional career. With that at stake, would any therapist-patient
ever enter treatment or honestly admit to sexual indiscretion? These
policy arguments were raised during the original *Tarasoff* debate.
In retrospect, even the harshest critics conceded that the duty to
warn is not as unmitigated a disaster as it once seemed (34). On
balance, confidentiality is generally favored, though silence must
be broken when, in individual cases, foreseeable harm is likely to
occur. As the *Tarasoff* limits of confidentiality become widely
known, patients will react accordingly. In the meanwhile, psychiatrists may wish to caution their patients that the therapeutic
relationship is not sacrosanct, thus conveying the essence of a
Miranda-like warning (35).

Conclusion

In this chapter, we have examined two types of situations in
which a psychotherapist learns of the sexual misconduct of a colleague. In the first case, a patient described her sexual involvement
with a former therapist. In the second, a therapist revealed his
sexual misconduct in his treatment with his own psychiatrist. Both
situations raise the question of whether the therapist has a duty to
protect his or her colleague's other patients from the danger of
sexual exploitation. There is little justification for applying the
Tarasoff doctrine to the first case. The therapist has no direct
evidence corroborating the accusation and a very narrow range of
effective actions. The therapist's most productive intervention would
be to assist the patient to file her own complaint with an ethics
committee or the state licensing board. However, the therapist-
patient who confesses to sexual misconduct confronts his psychiatrist with a traditional conflict between confidentiality and the
duty to protect third parties from harm. Even though the third
party is an adult who may not have resisted the sexual advances,
and the harm is psychological rather than physical, we believe the
psychiatrist has the ethical and perhaps legal responsibility to act.
In such instances, the treating psychiatrist can discharge his or her

duty to protect by notifying an ethics committee or the state licensing board. Ultimately, it is the licensing board that has the authority to restrict an abusive therapist's scope of practice in order to safeguard the public. By selectively breaching confidentiality, the treating psychiatrist has sought to safeguard the quality of life and preserve the integrity of the profession.

References

1. Kardiner SH, Fuller M, Mensh IN: A survey of physicians' attitudes and practices regarding erotic and nonerotic contact with patients. Am J Psychiatry 130:1077–1081, 1973
2. Holroyd JC, Brodsky AM: Psychologists' attitudes and practices regarding erotic and nonerotic physical contact with patients. Am Psychol 32:843–849, 1977
3. Freud S: Observations in transference-love (1915), in The Standard Edition of the Complete Psychological Works of Sigmund Freud, Vol 12. Translated and edited by Strachey J. London, Hogarth Press, 1958, pp 159–171
4. Bouhoutsos J, Holroyd J, Lerman H, et al: Sexual intimacy between psychotherapists and patients. Professional Psychology: Research and Practice 14:185–196, 1983
5. Feldman-Summers S, Jones G: Psychological impacts of sexual contact between therapists or other health care practitioners and their clients. J Consult Clin Psychol 52:1054–1061, 1984
6. Brown LS: Harmful effects of posttermination sexual and romantic relationships between therapists and their former clients. Psychotherapy 25:249–255, 1988
7. Herman JL, Gartrell N, Olarte S, et al: Psychiatrist-patient sexual contact: results of a national survey, II: psychiatrists' attitudes. Am J Psychiatry 144:164–169, 1987
8. Tarasoff v Regents of the University of California, 551 P2d 334, 17 Cal3d 425 (Cal Sup Ct 1976)
9. Mills MJ, Sullivan G, Eth S: Protecting third parties: a decade after *Tarasoff*. Am J Psychiatry 144:68–74, 1987
10. Kermani EJ, Drob SL: *Tarasoff* decision: a decade later dilemma still faces psychotherapists. Am J Psychotherapy 41:271–285, 1987
11. Beck JC (ed): The Potentially Violent Patient and the *Tarasoff* Decision in Psychiatric Practice. Washington, DC, American Psychiatric Press, 1985
12. Lipari v Sears, 497 FSupp 185 (D Neb 1980)

13. Petersen v Washington, 671 P2d 230, 100 (Wash 421 1983)
14. Stone AA: Vermont adopts *Tarasoff*: a real barn-burner. Am J Psychiatry 143:352–355, 1986
15. Eth S: The sexually active, HIV infected patient: confidentiality versus the duty to protect. Psychiatric Annals 18:571–576, 1988
16. American Psychiatric Association: AIDS policy: Confidentiality and disclosure. Am J Psychiatry 145:541, 1988
17. Pope KS: Research and laws regarding therapist-patient sexual involvement implications for therapists. Am J Psychother 40:564–571, 1986
18. Gartrell N, Herman J, Olarte S, et al: Psychiatrist-patient sexual contact: results of a national survey, I: prevalence. Am J Psychiatry 143:1126–1131, 1986
19. Simon RI: Sexual exploitation of patients: how it begins before it happens. Psychiatric Annals 19:104–112, 1989
20. Gartrell N, Herman J, Olarte S, et al: Reporting practices of psychiatrists who knew of sexual misconduct by colleagues. Am J Orthopsychiatry 57:287–295, 1987
21. Masters WH, Johnson VE: Principles of the new sex therapy. Am J Psychiatry 133:548–554, 1976
22. Stone AA: The legal implications of sexual activity between psychiatrist and patient. Am J Psychiatry 133:1138–1141, 1976
23. Gartrell N, Herman J, Olarte S, et al: Management and rehabilitation of sexually exploitive therapists. Hosp Community Psychiatry 39:1070–1074, 1988
24. Stone AA: Sexual misconduct by psychiatrists: the ethical and clinical dilemmas of confidentiality. Am J Psychiatry 140:195–197, 1983
25. Gutheil TG: Borderline personality disorder, boundary violations, and patient-therapist sex: medicolegal pitfalls. Am J Psychiatry 146:597–602, 1989
26. American Psychiatric Association: The Principles of Medical Ethics With Annotations Especially Applicable to Psychiatry. Washington, DC, American Psychiatric Association, 1985
27. Kilburg RR, Kaslow RW, VandenBos GR: Professionals in distress. Hosp Community Psychiatry 39:723–725, 1988
28. Vinson JS: Use of complaint procedures in cases of therapist-patient sexual contact. Professional Psychology: Research and Practice 18:159–164, 1987
29. California Business and Professions Code § 337
30. California Business and Professions Code § 728
31. Slovenko R: The therapist's duty to warn or protect third persons. Journal of Psychiatry and Law 16:139–209, 1988

32. Melella JT, Travin S, Cullen K: The psychotherapist's third-party liability for sexual assaults committed by his patient. Journal of Psychiatry and Law 15:83–116, 1987
33. Stone MH: Management of unethical behavior in a psychiatric hospital staff. Am J Psychother 29:391–401, 1975
34. Stone AA: Law, Psychiatry, and Morality. Washington, DC, American Psychiatric Press, 1984
35. Leong GB, Silva JA, Weinstock R: Ethical considerations of clinical use of Miranda-like warnings. Psychiatr Q 59:293–305, 1988

CHAPTER EIGHT

The HIV Antibody–Positive Patient

Kenneth Appelbaum, M.D.
Paul S. Appelbaum, M.D.

In early 1981, the first case of a new and unusual syndrome was diagnosed in the United States (1,2). Those afflicted with the condition—primarily homosexual men—experienced a breakdown in their bodies' immune systems, leaving them susceptible to a host of rare disorders. Almost overnight, doctors were confronted with a growing number of patients suffering from previously rare malignancies, opportunistic infections, and severe and refractory cases of common contagious illnesses. The condition came to be known as the acquired immunodeficiency syndrome, or AIDS. Within a few short years, AIDS progressed from an obscure disorder, largely limited to distinct subcultures within our society, to one that cuts across socioeconomic and life-style strata. Had the original locus of infection been in a different segment of society, recognition of the epidemic might have occurred even sooner.

This modern plague has spawned considerable concern within the medical, business, and lay communities. Researchers have isolated the causative virus, developed remarkably sensitive and specific laboratory tests for its identification, and revealed the sobering epidemiology of the infection. Ever-increasing numbers of lay and professional articles, books, journals, and conferences on AIDS have appeared. The Surgeon General's office has distributed educational materials on the topic to every household in the United States. Businesses and insurance companies are attempting to cope with the potentially enormous economic impact of the epidemic. Legislatures and courts are beginning to struggle with difficult questions of discrimination, public health measures, and liability.

The medical community is witnessing a shift from overcapacity to a shortage of hospital beds in areas hardest hit by the virus. The often-tacit assumption that every patient may elect to receive therapeutic interventions regardless of their expense or likely benefits has begun to be challenged, as critics contend that intensive care units and other scarce medical resources are turning into high-technology hospices. Meanwhile, a new generation of physicians is being trained at a time when little more than compassion and a willingness to assume the occupational risk of exposure can be offered to a growing number of young, but terminal, patients.

From the initial reports of AIDS in early 1981 through the end of August 1988, more than 72,000 cases were reported to the Centers for Disease Control (CDC), and it has been projected that by 1992, the cumulative total will be 365,000 cases (3). The CDC currently estimates that between 1 million and 1.5 million people in the United States are infected with the causative virus, human immunodeficiency virus (HIV) (3). Recent predictions are that 35–45% of infected individuals will develop either AIDS or AIDS-related complex (ARC) within 5–8 years of contracting the virus (4,5).

Although the virus has been isolated from most body fluids, there is no evidence that transmission through casual contact occurs. Blood, intimate sexual activity, perinatal exposure, and organ or tissue transplants are the vectors of infection, and the only means of prevention is through avoidance of exposure (6). There is no known cure for AIDS, and the syndrome to date is presumed uniformly fatal.

Conflicting Values: Confidentiality Versus Protection of Others

Along with the new syndrome have come new challenges for psychiatrists and other mental health professionals treating infected patients whose behavior places others at risk. To what extent are mental health professionals obligated—ethically or legally—to attempt to prevent persons in intimate contact with their patients from becoming infected with the virus? If action to protect third parties comes into conflict with therapists' traditional obligation to preserve the confidentiality of patients' disclosures, which value should take precedence?

The following case examples illustrate the range of situations in which these dilemmas arise.

Case Example 1

Ms. A, a 26-year-old, recently married woman, consults a psychiatrist with a chief complaint of anxiety. During the initial interview, Ms. A reveals that she is a former intravenous-drug abuser, and she recently learned that a friend with whom she had shared needles was diagnosed with AIDS. Ms. A is considering testing to determine her HIV antibody status, but she is fearful of the possible results. She informs the psychiatrist that her husband is a heavy drinker who has been physically abusive toward her. He is unaware of her history of drug abuse, and she believes that he would beat her if he learned of this or if he discovered that Ms. A was infected with the AIDS virus.

Should the psychiatrist encourage Ms. A to go ahead with testing? If she tests positive and refuses to reveal the result to her husband, should the psychiatrist do so? Must he tell her of his intention to do so before learning of the result of the test?

Case Example 2

Mr. B is a 35-year-old single, bisexual man who has been seen in individual psychotherapy for the past 4 months. While donating blood a year ago, he learned that he screened positive for HIV. Since that time, he has not been sexually active. He now informs his therapist that he has been dating a woman, who is also in her mid-30s, and they have begun talking of marriage and raising a family. They recently became sexually active, using condoms and foam for contraception. Mr. B is reluctant to tell her of his HIV status as he believes that doing so might destroy the relationship. He has a strong desire to have children, and he contends that the risk of transmission of the virus via heterosexual intercourse is very low.

What is the therapist's obligation to the patient's sexual partner?

Case Example 3

Ms. C is a 29-year-old single woman who supports herself through prostitution. She has a history of bipolar disorder and has just been involuntarily committed to a state psychiatric hospital with a diagnosis of an acute manic episode. She is grandiose, pressured, and hypersexual. During a previous admission 6 months ago, Ms. C had sexual intercourse with another patient in the hospital. She also tested positive for HIV at that time. Her ward psychiatrist has decided to inform other patients on the ward that Ms. C is infected with HIV and to warn them against sexual relations with her. He also intends to notify all hospital staff to avoid exposure to blood or body fluid from Ms. C because of her infection with the virus.

Is this behavior by the psychiatrist justified? Are there other ways in which the situation might be addressed?

Ethical Issues and Professional Guidelines

The moral dilemma arising with HIV-positive patients from the clash of obligations between maintaining patient confidentiality and protecting third parties has historical parallels. Earlier in this century, the medical community fiercely debated which imperative should be seen as paramount in instances where a physician knew that a patient was exposing another person to the risk of infection with a venereal disease. The resultant positions and their underlying rationales are similar to those expressed in the current controversy.

In perhaps simplistic fashion, some early twentieth century commentators contended for the absolute primacy of the "medical secret." Arguments supporting the maintenance of the "medical secret" were based on deontological principles, which hold that some acts are right and others are wrong independent of their consequences. The rights to privacy and autonomy, mainly derived from deontological theories, led some to conclude that "the reporting of any contagious malady [was] an outrage of individual right in the interest of the good of the majority" (7, p. 1203). The "shameful" nature of venereal disease and the fear that public disclosure of the patient's diagnosis "would cost him his position" in the community strengthened this deontological perspective, in-

voking the principle of nonmaleficence, or the duty to do no harm.
In addition, utilitarian concerns were voiced that if confidentiality
were compromised, "infected individuals would delay treatment
at the hands of the reputable physican and seek the aid of the quack
and the corner drugstore" (8, p. 312).

The opposite pole of the debate emphasized the physician's
beneficent obligation to take steps to prevent harm to individuals
unknowingly exposed to infection. This position was more open
to the recognition that any course of action would involve a violation of some fundamental principle in favor of another. With this
in mind, it was argued that the immorality of the patient's decision
to expose another to the risk of venereal disease weakened the
requirement of secrecy. If the patient were so "conscienceless,"
then the physician might "consider the criminal intent of this mon-
ster as entirely without the pale of professional protection" (9,
p. 61). A related form of analysis asserted that "if no other way
is open," the obligation of confidentiality is "less in degree than
the greater duty of saving life and preserving health" (10, p. 1209).

The AIDS epidemic has resurrected and intensified the historical dispute regarding the "medical secret." The burgeoning
number of professional organizations that have drafted guidelines
is testimony to the rapidity with which this issue has again been
thrust to the forefront of medical ethics. Our predecessors struggled without specific promulgations, but to the satisfaction of some
and the chagrin of others, contemporary medical associations have
begun to formulate policies.

The "AIDS Policy: Confidentiality and Disclosure" statement
of the American Psychiatric Association (APA) (11) defines the
circumstances under which confidentiality ethically may be breached.
It states that if "a physician has received convincing clinical information (the patient's own disclosure of test results or documented test records) that the patient is infected with HIV" and
the physician has "good reason to believe" that the patient's behavior is placing other persons "at continuing risk of exposure, it
is ethically permissible for the physician to notify an identifiable
person who the physician believes is in danger of contracting the
virus." Reporting of patients' names to "the appropriate public
health agency" is also deemed to be "ethically permissible." Patients should be informed in advance of limits on confidentiality

and "any breach of confidentiality should be a last resort, only after scrupulous attention has been given to all other alternatives." These alternatives include "the patient's agreement to terminate behavior that places other persons at risk of infection or to notify identifiable individuals who may be at continuing risk of exposure" (11, p. 541).

At the same time the preceding position was adopted, the APA Board of Trustees also approved the statement "AIDS Policy: Guidelines for Inpatient Psychiatric Units" (12). In part, this states, "If the patient engages in behavior likely to transmit the virus and there is a significant risk that such behavior cannot be controlled by other measures, then disclosure of a patient's infectious condition to other patients at risk is permissible." It also permits disclosure "to the appropriate staff only after discussions with the patient, if the physician determines that appropriate treatment of the patient requires such disclosure" (12). Delaying discharge due to the patient's engagement in high-risk behavior is described as "inappropriate" in the absence of other clinical indications for continued hospitalization.

Whereas the APA makes warning ethically permissible after other attempts to protect identifiable third parties have failed, the Council on Ethical and Judicial Affairs of the American Medical Association (AMA) appears to take a stronger stance, implying that there is an overriding obligation to warn (13). Specifically, they state

> Where there is no statute that mandates or prohibits the reporting of seropositive individuals to public health authorities and a physician knows that a seropositive individual is endangering a third party, the physician should (1) attempt to persuade the infected patient to cease endangering the third party; (2) if persuasion fails, notify authorities; and (3) if the authorities take no action, notify the endangered third party. (p. 1361)

In contrast, a joint position paper of the American College of Physicians and the Infectious Diseases Society of America (14) eschews taking a clear stance, stating

> The confidentiality of patients infected with HIV should be protected to the greatest extent possible, consistent with the duty to protect others and to protect the public health. (p. 466)

Although this position paper maintains that "the HIV-infected patient is obligated to inform his or her contacts," the physician is merely advised that "under some circumstances, the duty to inform will take precedence over the duty to protect confidentiality." In areas where the public health authorities have assumed the responsibility for informing individuals who are at risk, the physician's obligation would cease with the notification of those authorities. The "public health" component of this policy is especially worthy of note. Included in the duty to inform are past, as opposed to only ongoing, contacts with HIV-positive patients, through sex, shared needles, and blood or other body fluids.

The foregoing guidelines, as well as their discrepancies, highlight the ethical conflicts between the "medical secret" and the duty to protect third parties. The resolution of this dilemma can be approached from both deontologic and consequentialist perspectives. A deontologist must have some way of resolving the competing demands of confidentiality and beneficent protection of others. We believe that greater weight must be given to the protection of life than to even the serious but non-life-threatening harm that might result to the patient from disclosure. Studies of the pre-*Tarasoff* (15) behavior of therapists in related *Tarasoff*-like situations suggest that many would agree (16,17). Statutes and court cases requiring disclosure when lives of third parties are at risk indicate a growing societal consensus on this issue.

Consequentialist theories hold that the rightness of an act is determined mainly by its effects. The argument for maintaining confidentiality focuses on both the general benefits of maintaining societal trust in the privacy of the physician-patient relationship and the specific risks of discrimination and other adverse social consequences to the patient if sensitive information is disseminated. It is often argued that populations at high risk for infection with HIV will shun medical and mental health care if risk of disclosure of their HIV status exists. Concerns for the general effects of breaching confidentiality, while understandable, are rendered less compelling by experience with other exceptions to confidentiality. Statutes that mandate the reporting of contagious disease, child abuse, and gunshot injuries have existed for many years. There is no evidence that these requirements have either dissuaded patients from seeking treatment or significantly impaired the physician-patient relationship any more than *Tarasoff*-like obligations have hindered the utilization or practice of psychotherapy (18). As with the general duty to protect from violent harm, no data exist to support the assertion that HIV-positive patients will avoid contact with caregivers. In contrast, the potential for harm to those at risk for infection is obvious and real.

The potential for discrimination and harm to the patient must also be considered. Discrimination against HIV-positive persons occurs in housing, employment, access to insurance, and interpersonal contexts. Balanced against this is the risk of transmission of a life-threatening infection if the physician joins in the patient's silence. The facts that AIDS has no known cure, is almost universally fatal, and is readily preventable represent persuasive reasons for protecting third parties. We believe that the benefit from the preservation of life will generally exceed the harm of warning.

Some commentators contend that the balance of principles and consequences differs for members of high-risk groups (e.g., gay men or intravenous-drug abusers). It is argued that the demands of beneficence are lessened in cases where the third party knows, or should know, that he or she is engaging in "unsafe" sex or needle sharing. Alternatively, some people maintain that members of high-risk groups have received sufficient notice of the danger posed by their life-style so that specific warnings are unnecessary.

There are several difficulties with these stances. First, the assumption that these subcultures are medically sophisticated is unwarranted. Ignorance and misconceptions regarding the epidemiology of AIDS cut across the social spectrum. In addition, the use of denial is as prevalent in these groups as it is in any others. Some individuals do not consider themselves to be members of the high-risk population despite their life-styles (19). One should not surmise that a specific warning of personal peril would be superfluous. Misconceptions and denial can be corrected through direct contact with a physician, thus allowing the individual to make a more informed choice regarding continued exposure to HIV. The situation is analogous to progeny of the *Tarasoff* decision that have held that, even in cases where a third party was otherwise aware of a patient's threats, a therapist's warning is indicated to underscore the danger (20). Beyond that, declining to notify members of high-risk groups places them on an unequal footing relative to other members of the population and represents a subtle form of discrimination by promoting distinctions between "innocent" and "guilty" modes of contagion.

On balance, then, persuasive deontologic and consequentialist arguments can be made that physicians and mental health professionals have an ethical obligation to act to protect persons who might be infected by their patients.

Statutes and Case Law

Despite their differences, professional guidelines from medical organizations have generally agreed on the existence of a duty to protect third parties who are at risk for infection due to their contact with an HIV-positive patient. In contrast, the few state legislatures that have addressed this issue have reached antithetical positions, and case law on the question is limited. Law in this area, however, is developing rapidly.

Statutory situations regarding confidentiality and AIDS range from states that have no specific statutes addressing the issue (the majority at this point), to those with relatively strict confidentiality laws, to those that allow breaches under a broader set of circumstances (21). In states with restrictive statutes, unauthorized disclosures may constitute grounds for civil penalties; in at least three states, misdemeanor charges are possible. Medical emergencies may constitute an exception to confidentiality in some locales. In addition, some states with otherwise restrictive disclosure laws allow information to be divulged to a patient's spouse, to applicants for marriage licenses after mandatory testing, to jail or prison personnel, to persons who dispose of bodies, to persons who have provided emergency medical services to infected patients, and to past contacts after the patient's demise. In some cases, however, these exceptions are limited to documented cases of AIDS or ARC as opposed to cases of HIV infection without active illness, and they may cover only public health officials rather than medical or mental health personnel in general. Furthermore, the information that may be released often does not include the patient's name or identifying data. For example, those who dispose of bodies may be warned only to observe body-fluid precautions without being informed of the deceased's diagnosis, and emergency medical providers may be told of their exposure without revealing the patient's identity. (For a general review of state statutes, see the quarterly State Health Legislation report published by AMA.)

Case law regarding a health professional's legal obligations in this area is in a nascent state of development. A few cases are pending at the trial court level, including suits for failure to warn. Appellate decisions most likely will arise, but in the meantime, inferences drawn from related case law can provide some limited guidance.

The existence of a physician's legal duty to protect third parties who are placed at risk of harm by the physician's patient is supported by a long line of judicial decisions. The *Tarasoff* decision itself drew on precedents concerning patients with communicable diseases (22–25). In general, this line of decisions has limited the duty to identifiable third parties. The patient's spouse or fiancée or health care workers whose activities place them in danger of contracting the infection have been included in this category. In other cases, grounds for civil damage actions have been found in instances where either a physician failed to notify public health authorities of the existence of a reportable condition or a physician failed to inform the patient of the diagnosis, risk of transmission, and infection control measures. It is important to note, however, that where specific statutes exist, they will most likely supersede tenets developed in the common law.

In applying the foregoing information to a determination of legal obligations, additional factors are worthy of consideration. Some contend that for a defendant physician or mental health professional, a breach of confidentiality action is preferable to a wrongful death action. For a number of reasons, this may not be true in this instance. Even if the duty to protect is held to extend to HIV-related circumstances, major hurdles would remain in the way of a successful suit for failure to fulfill this duty. A finding of negligence due to failure to warn would be a necessary, but not sufficient, basis for liability. The plaintiff also would need to prove that some harm was inflicted and that the negligent omission of the warning was the proximate cause of that harm. This latter prerequisite could turn out to be an insurmountable obstacle in many legal actions for damages. The prolonged latency period between infection with HIV and the development of clinical symptoms will make it difficult to prove that transmission did not result from sexual or needle-sharing partners other than the patient or from contact with the patient occurring before the doctor's failure to warn.

Similarly, although reporting HIV and AIDS cases to public health authorities would mitigate the likelihood of a successful suit for failure to warn a third party, it would be difficult to show that noncompliance with reporting statutes was the proximate cause of transmission of the virus in view of the limited effectiveness of contact tracing in preventing individual cases. The defense also might argue that the plaintiff willingly assumed the risk of contagion by having intimate contact with the patient. The previously mentioned case precedents all involved infectious diseases that are transmissible through more casual contact. Therefore, successful suits for a breach of the duty to protect most likely will be rare.

In sum, the existence of a legal obligation to warn a person at risk of infection by a patient is unclear. Older case law would appear to support such an obligation, but recent decisions are lacking. Some states' statutes appear to preclude notification of parties at risk, although even here there are authorities who encourage disclosure on ethical grounds (26). Laws that permit disclosure to endangered persons, especially spouses, may prompt courts to make warnings mandatory when other protective steps are likely to be inadequate. At present, ethical obligations to protect third parties appear to be more compelling than possible legal duties.

Clinical Issues

Professional organizations that have published guidelines on AIDS confidentiality issues have tended to address the fundamental questions, whereas many of the nuances of management are left to the discretion of the individual practitioner. Details that are not fully explored include the process by which a patient's HIV status is determined, the definition of potential victims and the mechanisms for eliciting their identities, the hierarchy of possible responses in fulfilling the duty to protect, methods for monitoring the effectiveness of the intervention, and the nature of the warning when one is indicated. The following discussion will consider each of these issues in the clinical context, with particular reference to the APA guidelines.

Determining Patients' HIV Status

The APA policy requires the psychiatrist to inform a patient of the specific limits of confidentiality before inquiring about HIV status. Despite the acceptance of a duty to third parties, the APA appears to eschew the use of deceit in the elicitation of this information. The rationale for this stance may include the recognition that potential damage to the clinician-patient relationship resulting from breach of confidentiality would be unjustifiably compounded if the patient's HIV status was determined either through active duplicity or through the artifice of silence regarding the consequences of disclosure. Even the obligation to protect the life of an unwitting third party does not warrant deception. The necessity for a foundation of basic trust and respect within the therapeutic relationship is not negated by the existence of duties to persons outside the clinician-patient dyad.

The guidelines leave unspecified, however, whether information may be disclosed if it was acquired before a warning about the limits of confidentiality was given—as will often be the case. Although some actions in such circumstances may threaten the trust inherent in a therapeutic relationship, the value of protecting life must often take precedence. Careful discussion of the issues with the patient, of course, should be undertaken to minimize adverse effects on the therapist-patient relationship and may result in the patient's taking action that obviates the need for disclosure.

Another unanswered question is the extent to which the physician should advise the patient to pursue the determination of HIV serostatus. Encouraging testing goes beyond mere inquiry into existing test results. In our opinion, in most cases, a physician should recommend testing when a patient presents with a history of high-risk behavior. In Case Example 1, for instance, Ms. A would be counseled about the significance and potential implications of HIV test results and the limits of confidentiality regarding those results. She would be advised to undergo testing as knowledge of her serostatus would facilitate a more informed decision ` regarding her future behavior.

Identifying Persons at Risk

Once the patient's HIV status has been determined, the APA has little to say regarding the identification and definition of "other persons at risk of infection." The manner of their detection involves considerations similar to those raised by the process of eliciting the patient's serostatus. It would be no more appropriate to resort to guile at this phase of the inquiry than at any other. Discussion of the potential consequences of the disclosure of the patient's contacts is indicated before vigorous attempts to persuade the patient to modify his or her behavior or to identify those persons who are being placed at risk of infection. When contacts are not readily identifiable, the physician's ethical obligation to investigate further should be satisfied by attempts to elicit the information from the patient.

Although the definition of a person "at risk" might appear to be straightforward, it is, at times, a source of confusion. The three main modes of infection with the virus are sexual contact, inoculation with blood or its products, and perinatal exposure. Potential breaches of confidentiality primarily involve sexual partners and those who share needles with intravenous-drug users. Health care workers are also at risk from parenteral, mucous membrane, and nonintact skin exposures to the blood of HIV-positive patients. Identifiable persons who are in danger of contracting the virus, therefore, consist of individuals from these groups.

As previously noted, professional guidelines have differed as to whether the duty to warn third parties is limited to those "at continuing risk of exposure" (i.e., APA policy) or extends to past contacts (i.e., American College of Physicians and Infectious Diseases Society of America). Notification of prior exposure might prompt an individual to check his or her own serostatus. If positive, sexual and needle-sharing behavior could be modified and women might elect to forego future pregnancies. Disclosure to these persons would have to be based on an extension of the duty to protect to individuals at least once removed from the patient. This could become a process without end, as the physician assumes an obligation to warn the contacts of the patient's contacts. Limiting the physician's or mental health professional's duty to ongoing contacts appears to be both reasonable and practical, as it avoids saddling the physician with what is essentially a public health burden. Such contact tracing, however, might be a legitimate function of public health agencies.

Fulfilling a Duty to Protect

The limited options available with regard to past contacts highlight the wider range of alternatives in dealing with current behavior. *Tarasoff*-like obligations are often misconstrued as requiring solely a duty to warn. Although the initial 1974 decision of the California Supreme Court did frame the duty in this fashion, the court subsequently modified its position in 1976 and broadened the duty to warn to a duty to protect. In part, this involved a recognition that warning a third party might be the least effective and most noxious means of mitigating risk. In similar fashion, notification of contacts of HIV-positive patients may not be the first or best option to consider. APA suggests that psychiatrists "work with the patient . . . to obtain the patient's agreement to terminate behavior that places other persons at risk of infection" before considering a breach of confidentiality (11). Terminating the behavior eliminates the risk of contagion without compromising the patient's confidences. Compliance monitoring poses the major difficulty with this approach. The credibility of the patient's purported behavior change would require ongoing assessment and monitoring within the context of the physician-patient relationship. Although at times corroborative information may become available from other sources, assuming the role of private investigator is not generally indicated. If confirmation is deemed necessary, it may be sought discreetly and with the patient's awareness, though perhaps not always with the patient's consent.

Situations may arise where a patient is willing to modify, but not terminate, behavior that places others at risk of infection. In Case Example 2, Mr. B is practicing "safer" sex by using condoms. This decreases, but does not eliminate, the risk of contagion for his fiancée (nor does it solve the problem of their behavior after marriage when raising a family becomes an issue). It has been estimated that the risk of infection after a single act of unprotected intercourse with an HIV-positive partner is 1 in 500. The use of condoms reduces the likelihood of contagion to 1 in 5,000. After 500 sexual encounters, the estimated risk of infection is 2 in 3 without condoms and 1 in 11 with condoms (27). Mr. B's fiancée deserves the opportunity to decide for herself whether to chance this exposure. If, after appropriate education and counseling, Mr. B remains recalcitrant, the physician will need to consider alternatives to voluntary behavior changes.

If the patient will not agree to terminate high-risk behavior or if, in the words of the APA, "the physician has good reason to believe that the patient has failed to or is unable to comply with this agreement," then another option is a "report to the appropriate public health agency" (11). This should adequately fulfill the duty to third parties if the authorities are willing and able to conduct contact tracing and notification. However, in states where this is not the case, reporting will provide no protection for unwitting individuals who are at risk of infection and does not, in our view, constitute effective discharge of the ethical obligation.

In a limited number of instances, voluntary or involuntary psychiatric hospitalization may be indicated, but only where patients have mental disorders that warrant hospitalization. Similar to APA's proscription of delaying discharge "solely for quarantine or preventive detention," it would be inappropriate to pursue civil commitment for these purposes alone (12).

Warning Persons at Risk

Having exhausted other possible responses when confronted with a patient whose activity is placing an unsuspecting third party at risk for contagion with HIV, the physician is left with the question of whether the potential victim should be warned. The APA position is that it becomes "ethically permissible" for the psychiatrist to notify the third party only after the patient has refused or failed to terminate behavior that places others at risk or to notify, on his or her own, those individuals who are at continuing risk of exposure. The physician may warn only if the patient fails to do so. The scope of the warning is unspecified.

Ideally, the process of notification requires more than a mere statement that the individual is being exposed to potential contagion with HIV. As previously noted, widespread ignorance and misinformation regarding the epidemiology of AIDS exists. The significant distinction between "safer" sex techniques and complete avoidance of HIV-positive sexual partners may be misunderstood. Individuals also may assume improperly that, having already been exposed, it is too late for them to avoid infection. Alternatively, they may view themselves as being immune to the virus because they do not belong to the commonly perceived high-risk groups or for other mistaken reasons. Even if they are knowledgeable about the risks, a preliminary review of their options and where to go for further testing and counseling can be offered. The physician should be better equipped than even the most conscientious patient to tailor the notification to the unique educational needs of the individual. Furthermore, the warning may be more persuasive when it comes from a physician. For these reasons, information and referral from a physician is preferable to a warning from the patient. If the patient prefers, he or she could first broach the subject with the partner before contact by the physician. This would be the recommended approach in the case of Mr. B.

In inpatient settings, additional management options are available that generally make warnings unnecessary. Despite its sanction of disclosure of a patient's HIV status to other patients on a psychiatric unit, the APA policy acknowledges that this "is not a substitute for adequate clinical care and is usually inappropriate." In many cases, notifying other patients is the least effective and most deleterious alternative. The capacity of some psychiatric inpatients to utilize this information in a self-protective fashion is limited, and the breach of confidentiality is extensive. In contrast, clinical management of the infected patient's behavior, including possible use of isolation and restraint as recommended by the APA, may be efficacious in many cases. In the example of Ms. C, in addition to appropriate therapeutic interventions, the recommended response would include close observation during the manic episode to decrease the likelihood of sexual relations with other patients. This approach limits the danger to other patients while mitigating the harm to Ms. C. However, it probably requires that staff members be informed of the risk she presents.

In general, the risk of contagion to health care providers can be minimized by following CDC recommendations that "universal precautions" be followed with all patients regardless of their HIV serostatus (28,29). Although many workers in hospitals or residential settings (e.g., group homes) feel strongly about their right to know residents' HIV status, we believe that workers in these positions do not need to have this information—providing that body fluids, especially blood, are handled cautiously as a matter of routine. If it is elected to provide an additional alert to staff, in our opinion this should be accomplished by specifically designating the patient for blood and body-fluid precautions without identifying the patient's condition.

A final, and often overlooked option when responding to the duty to protect is to take no action at all. When effective alternatives do not exist or when the consequences of those alternatives are worse than doing nothing, then doing nothing becomes the appropriate response (30). At the time of Ms. C's discharge, for example, it was apparent that she intended to continue to practice her chosen profession despite attempts to dissuade her. Her treatment team was understandably concerned about the prospect that she would spread the virus. Nevertheless, continued civil commitment was rejected because her mania was in remission. Her decision to resume her prostitution was not due to her mental illness. Warning specific individuals was impractical. The police lacked the interest or resources to place her under surveillance, because many of the local streetwalkers are presumed to be infected with HIV. After consideration, it was concluded that there were no reasonable means of protecting her unidentifiable future contacts. A different dilemma might arise in the example of Ms. A, assuming that she undergoes screening for HIV and tests positive. The potential for her to be physically assaulted by her husband if he became aware of this might well preclude his notification.

Recommendations

In our opinion, the APA policies provide reasonable, albeit sparse, guidance for the physician confronted with an HIV-positive patient whose behavior is placing others at risk of infection. We endorse those guidelines, while offering the following additional recommendations regarding their implementation:

1. In most cases, physicians should advocate HIV laboratory testing for patients whose past histories and current behaviors suggest that third parties may be at risk of contagion.
2. Physicians should attempt, through direct and informed discussions with their patients, to identify third parties who are at risk of contagion.
3. Management options in outpatient settings include

   a. Termination of behavior that poses a risk of transmission of the virus
   b. Reporting to public health authorities if those authorities will conduct contact tracing and notification
   c. Hospitalization, when appropriate for the treatment of the patient's mental illness
   d. Warning and referral by the physician of the patient's contacts
   e. No action other than ongoing counseling of the patient, as indicated

4. Management options in inpatient settings include

   a. Appropriate treatment and adequate supervision to prevent the patient from engaging in behavior known to transmit HIV
   b. Adoption of "universal precautions" by staff

Summary

In the few years since its emergence, the AIDS epidemic has had a profound impact on modern society. The medical community has found itself confronted with myriad ethical dilemmas. A particularly thorny issue for mental health professionals involves the competing obligations to maintain patient confidentiality and to protect third parties. The historical debate regarding the "medical secret" has been resurrected by this modern plague, and professional guidelines, statutes, and case law have begun to address this question. In this chapter, we have attempted to review these topics and to explore clinical approaches to this problem. Specific recommendations that expand on current APA guidelines have been offered in the hope that they will assist in the mental health professional's decision making in this challenging area.

References

1. Centers for Disease Control: Pneumocystis pneumonia—Los Angeles. MMWR 30:250–252, 1981
2. Centers for Disease Control: Kaposi's sarcoma and Pneumocystis pneumonia among homosexual men—New York City and California. MMWR 30:305–308, 1981
3. Centers for Disease Control: Quarterly report to the domestic policy council on the prevalence and rate of spread of HIV and AIDS—United States. MMWR 37:551–559, 1988
4. Bayer R, Levine C, Wolf S: HIV antibody screening: an ethical framework for evaluating proposed programs. JAMA 256:1768–1774, 1986
5. Consensus Conference: The impact of routine HTLV-III antibody testing of blood and plasma donors on public health. JAMA 256:1778–1783, 1986
6. Friedland GH, Klein RS: Transmission of the human immunodeficiency virus. N Engl J Med 317:1125–1135, 1987
7. Keyes EL: The prenuptial sanitary guarantee. New York Medical Journal 85:1201–1204, 1907
8. Editorial: Shall venereal disease be reportable to the board of health. NY State J Med 11:311–312, 1911
9. Morrow PA: Social Diseases and Marriage. New York, Lea, 1904, p 61
10. Purrington WA: Professional secrecy and the obligatory notification of veneral diseases. New York Medical Journal 85:1206–1210, 1907
11. American Psychiatric Association: AIDS policy: Confidentiality and disclosure. Am J Psychiatry 145:541, 1988
12. American Psychiatric Association: AIDS policy: Guidelines for inpatient psychiatric units. Am J Psychiatry 145:542, 1988
13. Council on Ethical and Judicial Affairs: Ethical issues involved in the growing AIDS crisis. JAMA 259:1360–1361, 1988
14. Health and Public Policy Committee, American College of Physicians; and the Infectious Diseases Society of America: The acquired

immunodeficiency syndrome (AIDS) and infection with the human immunodeficiency virus (HIV). Ann Intern Med 108:460–469, 1988

15. Tarasoff v Regents of the University of California, 551 P2d 334, 131 Cal Rptr 14 (Cal Sup Ct 1976)

16. Wise TP: Where the public peril begins: a survey of psychotherapists to determine the effects of *Tarasoff*. Stanford Law Review 31:165–190, 1978

17. Givelber D, Bowers W, Blitch C: *Tarasoff*, myth and reality: an empirical study of private law in action. Wisconsin Law Review 443–497, 1984

18. Shuman DW, Weiner MF: The Psychotherapist-Patient Privilege: A Critical Examination. Springfield, IL, Charles C Thomas, 1987

19. Schorr JB, Berkowitz A, Cumming PD, et al: Prevalence of HTLV-III antibody in American blood donors. N Engl J Med 313:384–385, 1985

20. Jablonski v U.S., 712 F2d 391 (9th Cir 1983)

21. Matthews GW, Neslund VS: The initial impact of AIDS on public health law in the United States—1986. JAMA 57:344–351, 1987

22. Hofman v Blackmon, 341 So2d 752 (Fla App 1970)

23. Wojcik v Aluminum Co. of America, 183 NYS2d 351 (NY Supr Ct 1959)

24. Davis v Rodman, 227 SW 612 (Ark Supr Ct 1921)

25. Skillings v Allen, 173 NW 663 (Minn Supr Ct 1919)

26. Dickens BM: Legal limits of AIDS confidentiality. JAMA 259:3449–3451, 1988

27. Hearst N, Hulley S: Preventing the heterosexual spread of AIDS: are we giving patients the best advice? JAMA 259:2428–2432, 1988

28. Centers for Disease Control: Recommendations for prevention of HIV transmission in health-care settings. MMWR 36 (suppl 2S):1S–18S, 1987

29. Centers for Disease Control: Update: universal precautions for prevention of transmission of human immunodeficiency virus, hepatitis B virus, and other bloodborne pathogens in health-care settings. MMWR 37:377–388, 1988

30. Appelbaum PS: *Tarasoff* and the clinician: problems in fulfilling the duty to protect. Am J Psychiatry 142:425–429, 1985

CHAPTER NINE

Tarasoff and the Dual-Diagnosis Patient

Stephen J. Bartels, M.D.
Robert E. Drake, M.D., Ph.D.

Recent clinical research highlights the prevalence, clinical morbidity, and treatment difficulties of young patients dually diagnosed with schizophrenia and substance abuse (1). Clinical management of the dual-diagnosis patient is frequently complicated by violent and disruptive behavior (2–5). For the clinician treating this complex and often noncompliant patient, predicting and managing these behaviors are extremely difficult. The duties of the *Tarasoff* decision present a significant additional burden. Two out of three of the published *Tarasoff* cases that have found psychiatric liability for assaults by patients released from the hospital have involved dual-diagnosis patients (6,7).

At the heart of the *Tarasoff* decision is the directive to clinicians to assume increasing responsibility for predicting and preventing dangerous patient behavior. This obligation is based on the legal opinion that the relationship between clinician and patient has special characteristics that may abrogate the usual limits of confidentiality. In particular, *Tarasoff* mandates that the clinician has a duty to detect impending violence by the patient and to protect potential victims. This duty to protect may include warning the potential victim as well as exercising control over the patient in applying the civil commitment laws (6,8).

The clinician who attempts to comply with the directives of the *Tarasoff* decision is likely to find that the dual-diagnosis patient presents obstacles at every turn. Problems may occur in at least five areas: *1*) continuity of the treatment relationship, *2*) the capacity of the clinician to predict dangerousness, *3*) limitations of civil commitment laws, 4) the ability to identify and warn potential victims, and 5) the conflict between the duty to protect and the duty to maintain confidentiality.

First, the relationship between the outpatient clinician and the substance-abusing schizophrenic patient is often characterized by sporadic contacts, marginal engagement in treatment, and noncompliance (1). Ongoing symptom monitoring may be impossible. The therapeutic relationship is typically interrupted when the patient is actively abusing substances and is most likely to become violent. Nonetheless, the clinician continues to bear the burden of attempting to monitor and prevent dangerous behavior.

Second, even when the relationship is continuous, the clinician's capacity to predict dangerous behavior in schizophrenia is limited. The additional presence of substance abuse makes this task even more difficult. The schizophrenic patient who is abusing substances is known to be at greater risk to commit violent acts, yet guidelines for assessing dangerousness in the schizophrenic patient actively abusing substances have yet to be developed. There are virtually no data on predicting violence in the dual-diagnosis patient.

Third, the *Tarasoff* decision suggests that civil commitment laws can be effectively used to protect others from a patient at risk for violence. However, limitations in state statutes for involuntary commitment complicate this process when applied to the dual-diagnosis patient. These include requirements for a clear determination of imminent danger, the exclusion of hearsay evidence, and limits on the hospitalization of intoxicated patients. The last of these restrictions is ambiguous when applied to the dual-diagnosis patient. For example, New Hampshire criteria for involuntary hospitalization exclude "impairment primarily caused by . . . continuous or noncontinuous periods of intoxication caused by substances such as alcohol or drugs" (9, Section 2, X). The clinician is left to consider how this applies to the schizophrenic patient who becomes dangerously violent only when abusing substances.

Fourth, the duty to protect is clearest when potential victims can be identified and warned. Studies of violent acts by schizophrenic outpatients are extremely limited, but suggest that only a minority of victims can be identified in advance (10). Threats of violence indicate impending loss of impulse control that frequently represents a danger to others besides the named victim of the threat (11). Acts of violence are likely to be impulsive and related to physical proximity, rather than premeditated and directed at a preselected victim. This general and nonspecific danger to the community makes it difficult to identify who should be warned and when involuntary hospitalization is indicated.

Finally, the duty to protect may substantially compromise the treatment relationship. The inability to identify a specific potential victim may force the clinician to consider a broader warning to those who are most likely to come into contact with the patient. This might include warning the patient's family, social contacts, landlords, employers, and the police. However, excessive application of the duty to warn may substantially affect the current treatment relationship, the patient's future willingness to comply with treatment, the patient's remaining social supports, and ultimately, the clinician's ability to prevent dangerous behavior.

Each of these problems substantially complicates the treatment of the dual-diagnosis patient and potentially causes conflict with the duty to protect. The following case examples illustrate this ongoing tension between clinical and legal responsibilities.

Case Example 1

Frederich R is a 37-year-old, divorced, white male. He carries a diagnosis of schizophrenia and alcohol dependence and has been in and out of hospitals since his marriage dissolved 15 years earlier. After moving to our catchment area, he spent most of his time in the library working on plans to develop his own business. Mr. R was quite secretive about details, but his business plans sounded unrealistic to his caregivers. Mr. R lived alone in an apartment and was quite isolated since he was new to the area and made no efforts to meet anyone. He was cordial but distant during his required visits to the community mental health center (CMHC) and was actually quite wary of staff or patients who asked him about his personal life or past.

Some details of psychiatric history were known because Mr. R came out of the state hospital on a conditional discharge. This order contained his admission and discharge summaries and specified that he be required to participate in treatment for 6 months before attaining a regular discharge. Under the terms of a conditional discharge, he could be returned to the state hospital immediately for violating this agreement without meeting the usual commitment standards. His hospital records indicated that Mr. R had long-standing problems with a paranoid psychosis and alcoholism. On numerous occasions, when drinking, he had become disruptive, threatening, belligerent, and aggressive. His acts of aggression were usually directed at some stranger who Mr. R felt had wronged him. For example, his most recent hospitalization had occurred after he had slapped a restaurant patron who had inadvertently occupied a table that Mr. R felt was his. He had not injured anyone seriously. Mr. R's records also indicated that he denied his illness and was noncompliant with treatment.

Mr. R did comply with the terms of his conditional discharge for the 6 months that it was in effect. He received 1 cc of fluphen-azine decanoate im every 2 weeks, met with his case manager weekly, attended a patient education group weekly, and attended Alcoholics Anonymous three times a week. Although he acknowl-edged his problem with alcohol, he continued to deny psychiatric illness and declined offers of involvement beyond that required by his conditional discharge. As soon as the conditional discharge ex-pired, he asked to be taken off fluphenazine decanoate. His paranoia gradually increased over 2 months thereafter, at which point he dropped out of treatment entirely. Our many efforts to anticipate future problems and to understand prodromal symptoms were to no avail, as he continued to deny symptoms even as they worsened. Further efforts at outreach were angrily dismissed; Mr. R made it clear that he wanted no further contact with our staff. During this time and before, he also was adamant that we respect his right to confidentiality and have no contact with anyone in the community about him.

The next few months were distressing. Our staff observed Mr. R several times in restaurants when he was involved in angry al-tercations with other patrons and waitresses. We heard that he was banned from the local transport bus and several restaurants. His landlord called to inform us that Mr. R was drinking heavily and would soon lose his apartment. Staff felt that they could not share information about Mr. R with people from the community. Further efforts by our staff to engage Mr. R resulted in his refusal to answer his telephone or door. History suggested that it was just a matter of time before an assault would occur, but we had no idea when that might happen. Because we had no direct evidence of threatening behavior (or even of Mr. R's condition), we were unable to know exactly when he was to become "imminently dangerous" and thus meet criteria for involuntary hospitalization. Would it be this week or in 3 months? How could we intervene to protect the public and Mr. R himself from the consequences of his behavior? Because there was no identified victim, could we inform the police or anyone else about the potential for danger? When people from the community (such as storekeepers and the landlord) called us, could we acknowledge that we knew Mr. R or share information about him? Staff members were divided on these issues.

We decided to try to channel all calls from the community to the police directly, with the hope that Mr. R would be apprehended and brought in for a psychiatric evaluation before committing a dangerous act. We informed the police that some of our patients who were not taking medications were in an agitated state that might lead to dangerousness and that we would be willing to evaluate at any time such persons who came to their attention. Unfortunately, however, Mr. R was apprehended by the police only after committing a violent assault on a female motorist who blew her car horn at him for jaywalking in front of her car. He was intoxicated and quite psychotic at the time of the incident. He was then evaluated and judged dangerous on the basis of current clinical state and past history. He returned to the state hospital for another period of forced medications and another conditional discharge. On discharge from the hospital, he moved out of our catchment area. We were left with many questions about our failure to prevent the violent episode that led to readmission.

Case Example 2

Sam K is a 35-year-old man with a 10-year history of paranoid schizophrenia complicated by alcohol and polydrug abuse with multiple involuntary hospitalizations for bizarre and threatening behavior. When we first saw him at our CMHC 4 years ago, he was living at his parents' home where they had adapted a garage into living quarters. Although he sporadically attended our day treat-

ment program, he spent days at a time drinking beer and ingesting bottles of over-the-counter stimulants consisting of ephedrine-containing cold medications and caffeine tablets. His parents reported that Mr. K frequently became extremely agitated and paranoid, and on several occasions smashed all of the furniture in his room, claiming that listening devices had been planted there by the government to monitor his activity.

After one of these episodes of destructive behavior, Mr. K was involuntarily hospitalized for 6 months at the state hospital. Shortly after admission, he assaulted a male attendant because of hallucinations that told him he was going to be "sexually abused." He was placed on a moderate dose of fluphenazine with rapid resolution of his threatening and agitated behavior. Although he persistently experienced background auditory hallucinations and mild residual paranoid ideation, he became a model patient who was well liked by all of the staff. Nonetheless, his parents refused to accept him back into their home. After extensive planning, he was discharged to one of the CMHC group homes on intramuscular fluphenazine decanoate in conjunction with assertive case management, substance abuse counseling, and day treatment.

The staff at the group home initially remarked that Mr. K was extremely pleasant and cooperative and found it hard to believe that he had the potential to be violent. After several months, this impression changed when he once again became extremely agitated, hostile, and paranoid after abusing large quantities of over-the-counter stimulants and alcohol. During this time, he once again developed paranoid ideas and auditory hallucinations about sexual abuse. He believed that certain people driving red cars were behind this conspiracy. Eventually, he was again hospitalized after slashing the tires of several cars in town.

This pattern recurred several times in the months that followed and included two inpatient stays on an alcohol treatment unit. Although Mr. K generally complied with his intramuscular fluphenazine, he repeatedly abused alcohol and stimulants with concomitant exacerbations of his psychotic symptoms and dangerous behavior. In the context of one of these episodes, he suddenly threw a kitchen knife at a staff member in the group home and narrowly missed, resulting in yet another hospitalization.

The group home staff felt that Mr. K was potentially dangerous whenever he abused alcohol or over-the-counter medications, yet felt powerless to predict imminent dangerousness or to control his substance abuse. Commitment laws would not support the mere presence of substance abuse as a valid reason for involuntary hospitalization. Furthermore, in view of the frequent pattern of abuse, automatic rehospitalization for substance abuse did not seem practical. Frustrated, the staff decided to banish Mr. K from the supervised group home program until he could control his substance abuse problem.

After discharge from the hospital, Mr. K moved into a low-income boarding house. He later destroyed his room during an episode of substance abuse and acute paranoia resulting in criminal charges and eviction. The terms of probation included authorization to administer fluphenazine and disulfiram involuntarily. In addition, the CMHC became Mr. K's payee and restricted his use of funds for alcohol and over-the-counter medications. Nonetheless, Mr. K was able to borrow money from fellow patients and friends. Banned from all local housing, he no longer had a stable place to live and was relegated to sleeping on friends' floors or living out in the woods in a tent.

Although the staff at the day hospital felt that Mr. K was no longer abusing alcohol and generally seemed more stable, they suspected that he continued to obtain money from friends to purchase over-the-counter stimulant medications. At times he appeared more agitated, pressured, and paranoid, but did not indicate any overt signs of threatening or dangerous behavior. Plans were made to monitor him through regular drug screens.

In the midst of this assessment, Mr. K failed to appear for treatment over several days and could not be located. Staff eventually notified the police and expressed concerns about his past behaviors. The possibility of recurrent dangerous behavior was considered, but there were no identified potential victims. In spite of a general agreement that Mr. K was likely to become more delusional and to present a danger to the community, the staff felt that they lacked the means and indications for any further intervention.

After a 1-week absence, Mr. K resurfaced having engaged in a rampage of destructive and dangerous behavior. Believing that the conspiracy against him now included most of the town, he attacked parked cars with an ax in the middle of the night and set fire to several garages. Acutely paranoid and agitated, he finally wandered out into an intersection, threw the ax through the windshield of a slowly moving car, and seriously injured the driver.

The local newspaper ran this story on its front page and described Mr. K as a patient actively in treatment at the CMHC. A spokesperson for the police noted that the patient had a known history of violent behavior and implied that the case had been mismanaged. In discussing the outcome, staff expressed feelings of frustration, anger, and demoralization. They felt that the community was holding them responsible for the violence and suggested that the agency refuse to provide further treatment for Mr. K after discharge from the hospital. The administrators of the clinic privately voiced concerns of liability and braced themselves for legal and political repercussions.

These case examples illustrate many of the dilemmas facing the clinician responsible for the assessment and treatment of the dual-diagnosis patient. The added responsibilities implied by the *Tarasoff* decision exceed the limits of what is known about alcohol and drug abuse in schizophrenia, as well as what is known about predicting violence in this population. The clinician's ability to act responsibly is further impaired by social, legal, and clinical standards that provide exceptions for the consequences of behavior related to substance abuse. This is directly translated into different philosophies of prescribing and mandating treatment for substance-abuse disorders. In the section that follows, we summarize the literature on violence and substance abuse in schizophrenia as it applies to the *Tarasoff* decision.

Violence and Substance Abuse in Schizophrenia

A limited, but cogent, literature points toward high rates of substance abuse in schizophrenia and a clear link between substance abuse and violence. Our knowledge of the violent dual-diagnosis patient derives from research on aggression and substance abuse in schizophrenia.

Phenomenology of Violence in Schizophrenia

Most of the data on aggressive behavior in schizophrenia come from retrospective hospital chart reviews. Patients with schizophrenia are responsible for the majority of violent acts on psychiatric inpatient units. Eight to 45% of schizophrenic inpatients commit an aggressive act during their hospitalization (12–15). Most are young (12,15), male (16), and hospitalized involuntarily (16) and have a prior history of violent behavior (12,15,17,18). They are generally more acutely psychotic with prominent thought disorder characterized by disorganization (19–21).

Most aggressive acts occur shortly after admission, with the lowest rates of aggression occuring among those who have been in the hospital the longest (18). Low serum levels of antipsychotic medication at the time of admission (20) and neuroleptic-induced side effects such as akathisia (22) have been associated with violent behaviors. Neurological abnormalities have also been identified as risk factors for assaultive behavior in addition to past histories of violent crime, violent suicide attempts, and a deviant family environment in childhood (17). In one of the few investigations considering dangerous behaviors and substance-abuse histories of schizophrenic inpatients, Yesavage and Zarcone (23) found that a past history of blackouts and assaultiveness while drinking was related to subsequent assaultive behavior in the hospital. The extent to which inpatient violence is directly related to either toxic or withdrawal effects of substance abuse has not been studied.

One retrospective study of violence over the course of schizophrenic illness supports the association of violence with disorganized thinking and impulsivity. Planansky and Johnston (24) found that 10% of patients with schizophrenia were assaultive at some time during their lifetime. Disorganized thinking, nonsystematized delusions and hallucinations, and paranoid subtype were associated with verbal and physical attacks. It was unusual for violence to occur as an organized, premeditated act stemming from psychotic illness. Of those patients with a history of assaults, only 12% were responding to command hallucinations, and 5% were responding to systematized delusions compelling them to kill. For these patients, targets of violence tended to be familiar persons, rather than strangers.

In summary, studies of the phenomenology of violent behavior in schizophrenia suggest two general patterns. Uncommon, but highly dangerous, is the schizophrenic patient with a systematized paranoid delusion who commits a planned act of violence that targets a specific person in the patient's life. Although this patient is impaired in reality testing, he or she is typically intact enough to execute a complex plan. Such patients account for a high proportion of murders by psychiatric patients. In contrast, the majority of violent acts are commited by the patient who becomes assaultive in the context of an agitated or disorganized psychotic state. In this instance, violence is often unfocused, less planned, and generally less lethal (10).

Substance Abuse and Violence in Schizophrenia

Substance abuse is a common codiagnosis among schizophrenic patients in the community. Approximately one-half or more of young schizophrenic patients in the community actively abuse alcohol or other drugs (5,25). This use of psychoactive substances is associated with increased psychiatric symptoms (2,26,27), unstable clinical course (28), increased hospitalization (25,29), and suicidal (30) or assaultive behavior (4,5,27).

Studies exclusively focusing on outpatients clearly link substance abuse with increased rates of arrest and legal difficulties. In one study of substance-abusing psychiatric patients (two-thirds diagnosed with schizophrenia), Safer (5) found that 70% had law violations, compared to 15% in the nonabusing group. Zitrin et al. (31) reported similar findings in a study of arrest rates of schizophrenic patients over the 2 years before and 2 years after hospitalization from Bellevue Hospital. Of the 10% who had been arrested for violent offenses, one-half had a history of alcohol abuse, and one-fifth had been drug dependent and alcoholic.

Investigations of disruptive behavior by psychiatric patients in the community also show a clear link to substance abuse. Richardson et al. (32) found that 45% of schizophrenic patients have a history of violence and drug abuse, compared to 20% who have histories of violence without drug abuse. Drake et al. (25) found that hostile, threatening behavior was associated with alcohol use. McCarrick et al. (4) found that use of alcohol or other drugs was associated with disruptive behavior in the home and the community. Furthermore, the combination of alcohol and other drugs substantially increased disruptive behaviors when compared with alcohol or drugs alone.

The Clinician's Ability to Predict Violence

The clinician evaluating a dual-diagnosis patient has few guidelines for estimating the likelihood of violent behavior. We know of no studies that specifically identify factors associated with imminent violence in substance-abusing schizophrenic patients. The most difficult clinical decisions usually occur when the patient is out in the community and is known to present a potential threat to the safety of others.

The clinician who elicits a history of a paranoid delusion and a well-planned act of violence has the information necessary to warn potential victims and to arrange for involuntary hospitalization. However, the schizophrenic patient who is actively abusing substances more commonly fits the description of the disorganized, incoherent, and threatening patient. This patient has an increased risk of violence, yet the imminence, means, and victim are largely unpredictable. In these situations, the clinician is without clear guidelines as to *when* to exercise the duty to protect and *whom* to protect.

Researchers have been unable to agree on symptoms that reliably predict violent behaviors. For example, the significance of paranoid symptoms and hostility in predicting threatening and assaultive behavior in schizophrenia is controversial. Of seven studies examining paranoid versus nonparanoid subtypes, four found that violent behavior was more common in paranoid patients, two found that nonparanoid patients were more violent, and one found no difference between these types (10). Similarly, a relationship between expressed hostility and subsequent violence has been found by some investigators (18,33) but not by others (19). When visible cues do not precede violent acts, the assaultive patient is likely to be more thought disordered and withdrawn, in contrast to the hostile, suspicious, agitated patient whose risk of potential violence may be more identifiable (21).

Models and scales for predicting violence in psychiatric inpatients have generally been no more than 33% accurate (18), although recent studies suggest improvement in prediction (17,18). For example, the prediction of short-term dangerousness may be surprisingly accurate when patients have been clearly identified for emergency civil commitment by a hospital emergency service. McNeil and Binder (34) found that approximately two-thirds of those committed due to dangerousness engaged in violent behavior in the first 72 hours of hospitalization. In a later report, these same authors found that specific threats of violence made by schizophrenic patients within the 2 weeks before admission were strongly correlated with subsequent physical assaults and seclusion in the first 3 days of hospitalization (11). They concluded that threats of violence indicate an increased risk of dangerousness that extends beyond the intended victim and recommend a broad interpretation of the *Tarasoff* duty to protect that considers the risk to the general public.

Unfortunately, the outpatient clinician is often confronted with more ambiguous signs of potential dangerousness that neither involve a specific threat nor meet the criteria for involuntary hospitalization. Schizophrenic patients who abuse substances are often chronically disorganized, hostile, and noncompliant with treatment (25). It remains to be proven that violent behavior can be accurately predicted in schizophrenia, let alone in schizophrenic outpatients who have an active substance-abuse problem.

Court Decisions Relevant to the Dual-Diagnosis Patient

Beck (6) has reviewed recent court decisions in *Tarasoff*-type cases, including several that directly apply to the dual-diagnosis patient. There are now three published inpatient-release cases in which psychiatrists have been found liable: two involved dual-diagnosis patients (7). In the first of these two cases, *Davis v. Lhim* (35), a schizophrenic man with a history of heroin addiction and alcohol abuse killed his mother 2 months after discharge from the state hospital. There was no evidence of dangerousness at the time of discharge. The evidence supporting a finding of foreseeable violence was based on an emergency room note 2 years earlier that documented the patient threatening his mother for money. In the second case, *Petersen v. Washington* (36), a patient with schizo-phrenia and a history of phencyclidine (PCP) abuse injured a woman 5 days after discharge from the hospital while driving under the influence of drugs. The patient's psychotic symptoms had appeared to fully resolve during the 4-week hospitalization, yet the court found that the treating psychiatrist was negligent in failing to seek additional confinement based on "a duty to take reasonable pre-cautions to protect anyone who might foreseeably be endangered by the patient's drug-related mental problems" (36, p. 236).

Beck notes that violence was not clearly foreseeable in either case and that neither patient was considered committable at the time of discharge. Nonetheless, the courts found that a duty to seek additional confinement was indicated. Furthermore, each de-cision specifically mentioned the patient's substance-abuse problem as an important factor in estimating the patient's potential dan-gerousness.

In contrast, Beck describes a different outcome in a case where an outpatient with paranoid schizophrenia and alcoholism injured a married couple while driving under the influence of alcohol. In *Hasenei v. U.S.* (37), the patient had a known history of alcohol-related violence and had recently resumed drinking along with discontinuing his antipsychotic medications. The patient refused hospitalization 12 days before the accident and was judged by his clinicians not to be committable. In this case, the court did not find that the outpatient relationship provided sufficient control over the patient to create a duty to protect and similarly did not find a basis for medical certainty of the patient's dangerousness. This case supports Beck's conclusion that the courts may recognize a different degree of control for outpatient and inpatient clinicians.

Despite the lack of consensus on basic standards of care for the dual-diagnosis patient, and despite the adherence to usual stan-dards of care, vastly different decision were reached by the courts in these three cases (6). These discrepancies may in part reflect the considerable disagreement that exists regarding the clinician's abil-ity to predict dangerousness among dual-diagnosis patients.

Conclusions

Substance abuse is a common problem in schizophrenia and results in significant morbidity. Even moderate use can significantly exacerbate symptoms. The substance-abusing schizo-phrenic has an increased risk of violence, but the obstacles to fulfilling the duty to protect are considerable. These include patient noncompliance, the timing and pattern of aggression, limits on involuntary treatment, and the clinician's duty to maintain confidentiality.

Identifying and warning potential victims in the community is particularly difficult because violence by dual-diagnosis patients is usually disorganized and random. *Tarasoff*-type cases that have found liability for violence committed by substance-abusing schizophrenic patients suggest an ability to predict dangerousness that is not supported by the scientific literature. In fact, little is known about the prediction and management of violent behavior in the dual-diagnosis patient. Further research is necessary to develop guidelines for determining danger, mandating involuntary treatment, and informing those at risk from patient violence in a way that balances the patient's right to confidentiality with the obligation to protect others.

References

1. Ridgely SM, Osher FC, Talbot JA: Chronic Mentally Ill Young Adults With Substance Abuse Problems: Treatment and Training Issues. Baltimore, MD, University of Maryland, 1987
2. Alterman A, Erdlen F, McLellan AT, et al: Problem drinking in hospitalized schizophrenic patients. Addict Behav 5:273–276, 1980
3. Drake RE, Wallach MA: Dual diagnosis among the chronic mentally ill. Hosp Community Psychiatry 40:1041–1046, 1989
4. McCarrick AK, Manderscheid RW, Bertolucci DE: Correlates of acting-out behaviors among young adult chronic patients. Hosp Community Psychiatry 36:848–853, 1985
5. Safer DJ: Substance abuse by young adult chronic patients. Hosp Community Psychiatry 38:511–514, 1987
6. Beck JC: The therapist's legal duty when the patient may be violent. Psychiatr Clin North Am 11:665–679, 1988
7. Beck JC: Personal communication, 1989
8. Appelbaum PS: Legal aspects of violence by psychiatric patients, in Psychiatry Update: American Psychiatric Association Annual Review, Vol 6. Edited by Hales RE, Frances AJ. Washington, DC, American Psychiatric Press, 1987, pp 549–566

9. NH Rev Stat Ann (RSA) 135–C:2, X 135–C:27 et seq, 1987
10. Krakowski M, Volavka J, Brizer K: Psychopathology and violence: a review of the literature. Compr Psychiatry 27:131–148, 1986
11. McNeil DE, Binder RL: Relationship between preadmission threats and later violent behavior by acute psychiatric patients. Hosp Community Psychiatry 40:605–608, 1989
12. Karson C, Bigelow LB: Violent behavior in schizophrenic inpatients. J Nerv Ment Dis 175:161–164, 1987
13. Shader RJ, Jackson AH, Harmatz JS, et al: Patterns of violent behavior among schizophrenic inpatients. Diseases of the Nervous System 38:13–16, 1977
14. Fotrell E: A study of violent behavior among patients in psychiatric hospitals. Br J Psychiatry 136:216–221, 1980
15. Tardiff K, Sweillam A: Assaultive behavior among chronic inpatients. Am J Psychiatry 139:212–215, 1982
16. Rossi AM, Jacobs M, Monteleone M, et al: Characteristics of psychiatric patients who engage in assaultive or other fear-inducing behaviors. J Nerv Ment Dis 174:154–160, 1986
17. Convit A, Jaeger J, Lin SP, et al: Predicting assaultiveness in psychiatric inpatients: a pilot study. Hosp Community Psychiatry 39:429–434, 1988
18. Kay SR, Wolkenfeld F, Murrill LM: Profiles of aggression among psychiatric patients. J Nerv Ment Dis 176:539–557, 1988
19. Yesavage JA, Werner PD, Becker J, et al: Inpatient evaluation of aggression in psychiatric patients. J Nerv Ment Dis 169:299–302, 1981
20. Yesavage JA: Correlates of dangerous behavior by schizophrenics in hospital. J Psychiatr Res 18:225–231, 1984
21. Tanke ED, Yesavage JA: Characteristics of assaultive patients who do and do not provide visible clues of potential violence. Am J Psychiatry 142:1409–1413, 1985
22. Herrera JN, Sramek JJ, Costa JF, et al: High potency neuroleptics and violence in schizophrenia. J Nerv Ment Dis 176:558–561, 1988
23. Yesavage JA, Zarcone V: History of drug abuse and dangerous behavior in inpatient schizophrenics. J Clin Psychiatry 44:259–261, 1983
24. Planansky K, Johnston R: Homicidal aggression in schizophrenic men. Acta Psychiatr Scand 55:65–73, 1977
25. Drake RE, Osher FC, Wallach MA: Alcohol use and abuse in schizophrenia: a prospective community study. J Nerv Ment Dis 177:408–414, 1989
26. Negrete JC, Knapp WP: The effects of cannabis use on the clinical

condition of schizophrenics. Natl Inst Drug Abuse Res Mongr Ser 67:321–327, 1986

27. Knudsen P, Vilmar T: Cannabis and neuroleptic agents in schizophrenia. Acta Psychiatr Scand 69:162–174, 1984

28. Kesselman MS, Solomon J, Beaudett M, et al: Alcoholism and schizophrenia, in Alcoholism and Clinical Psychiatry. Edited by Solomon J. New York, Plenum, 1982, pp 69–80

29. Carpenter MD, Muligan JC, Bader IA, et al: Multiple admissions to an urban psychiatric center: a comparative study. Hosp Community Psychiatry 36:1305–1308, 1985

30. Noreik K: Attempted suicide and suicide in functional psychoses. Acta Psychiatr Scand 52:81–106, 1975

31. Zitrin A, Hardesty AS, Burdock EI, et al: Crime and violence among mental patients. Am J Psychiatry 133:142–149, 1976

32. Richardson MA, Craig TJ, Haugland MA: Treatment patterns of young schizophrenic patients in the era of deinstitutionalization. Psychiatr Q 57:104–110, 1985

33. Werner PD, Yesavage JA, Becker MT, et al: Hostile words and assaultive behavior on an acute inpatient psychiatric unit. J Nerv Ment Dis 171:385–387, 1983

34. McNeil DE, Binder RL: Predictive validity of judgments of dangerousness in emergency civil commitment. Am J Psychiatry 144:197–200, 1987

35. Davis v Lhim, 335 NW2d 481, 124 (Mich App 291 1983)

36. Petersen v Washington, 671 P2d 230, 100 (Wash 421 1983)

37. Hasenei v U.S., 541 FSupp 999 (D Md 1982)

CHAPTER TEN

Posttraumatic Stress Disorder and the Duty to Protect

Landy F. Sparr, M.D., M.A.
David J. Drummond, Ph.D.

Although the term *posttraumatic stress disorder* (PTSD) is new, the definition and the description of the disorder draw on earlier concepts of gross stress reaction and traumatic neurosis (1). The DSM-III and DSM-III-R criteria for PTSD have been investigated, and there is empirical support for both definitions (2–4). The major unifying features of PTSD, as described in DSM-III and DSM-III-R, are *1*) the occurrence of a severe stressor, *2*) the reexperiencing of the traumatic event, *3*) numbing of responsiveness and/or persistent avoidance of stimuli associated with the trauma, *4*) cognitive dysfunctions, and *5*) autonomic reactions to reminders of the traumatic event. The lumping of various stress disorders such as reactions to natural disasters, severe burns, or rape into a single diagnostic category had the advantage of simplifying and consolidating diverse studies of catastrophic stress. Nevertheless, it has been suggested that different stressors and different circumstances may produce different syndromes. For example, combat-related PTSD may be different from PTSD after other trauma. Lindy et al. (5) found wide group variation when comparing Hopkins Symptom Checklist scores for survivors of different types of trauma. Also, children present a somewhat different clinical picture after experiencing trauma than adults (6). In this chapter, we will primarily consider combat-related PTSD.

Some investigators, while validating DSM-III criteria in general, have also found evidence for additional specific features, for example, depression (7) or an avoidant subtype (8). Others, arguing that it is false to separate particular facets from the nexus of postwar maladjustment, have advocated a much broader definition of PTSD to include such behavior patterns as nomadism, antisociality, and substance abuse (9–11).

Consequently, when DSM-III-R was introduced in 1987, there was an attempt to broaden and refine the diagnosis of PTSD. For instance, among Vietnam veterans, various studies have found rage or anger to be a feature of PTSD (10–12). As a result, irritability or outbursts of anger, formally a DSM-III associated feature of PTSD, was included in DSM-III-R as a cardinal feature. Other new symptoms were added to the DSM-III-R PTSD section that concerns numbing of responsiveness. Guilt, a symptom that has not been empirically supported, was dropped.

Presumably, the largest single cohort of individuals suffering from symptoms of PTSD are Vietnam veterans; a conservative estimate is 500,000 to 750,000 veterans with the disorder (13). Often this primarily male population has participated in or witnessed wartime acts of violence that have been shown to play an evocative role in the later development of PTSD. For instance, exposure to combat or its consequences in Vietnam (e.g., by field hospital nurses, graves registration workers) has been the factor that most often correlates with postwar psychological distress in clinical (14,15), compensation-seeking (16), and community samples (17–19). The civilian arrest rate among Vietnam veterans with heavy combat exposure has been shown to be three times the rate among veterans who experienced light or no combat (17). Other factors related to military service may be associated with subsequent adjustment, e.g., the individual's perception of the meaning of combat (20,21), the degree of personal responsibility for combat-related tragedies (22), the general pattern of conduct during duty (15), and the mode of discharge after combat (23). Participation in atrocities confers especially high risk for PTSD (9). Secondary avoidance mechanisms (24) and postwar family and social supports may also influence symptoms of PTSD (23,25,26).

Although violence, paranoia, and even criminal behavior have been linked with combat-related PTSD, they are not part of the diagnostic criteria and are not prima facie evidence for PTSD as some would contend. Archer and Gartner (27) studied postwar homicide rate changes in 50 warring nations and 30 noncombatant control nations. Most of the combatant nations in the study experienced substantial postwar increases in their rates of homicide. These increases did not occur among the control group of noncombatant nations. They concluded that the model of the violent veteran, although difficult to disconfirm, could not be a sufficient explanation for postwar homicide rate increases. They suggested that the changes were more related to overall societal legitimation of violence during and after war.

Paranoia

Terror was common in the Vietnam War—a war in which the enemy was invisible and there was brutalization on both sides. Shatan (28) spoke of paranoid hyperalertness being encouraged in basic training. This stance was adaptive in combat but maladaptive elsewhere. Smith (29) concludes that survival was the buzzword in Vietnam. Complete safety was elusive and therefore combat paranoia was "endemic." The combat marine (the "Green Machine"), who was supposed to be cold, tough, and efficient, denied or suppressed feelings of guilt, fear, and grief (30). The training process required two things of the successful soldier: a constant proving of adequacy via dominance and aggression and a denial of intimacy. Eisenhart (31) has remarked that even though one objective was the allegiance of the Vietnamese population, little or no effort was made to familiarize soldiers with Vietnamese culture. Instead, terms such as "gook" were promoted that helped to define the Vietnamese as less than human. Kelman (32) has commented extensively on the role of dehumanization in the perpetuation of violence against fellow human beings. Egendorf (33) remembered that "the military managed to stir up the most extreme resentments and rage we had ever felt" (p. 119).

Hendin (34) has described paranoia after war trauma in which civilian life is treated as an extension of combat. For veterans with this adaptation, the meaning of the combat experience is usually linked to an angry response to their own vulnerability. Anger serves the function of helping to overcome fear and deny guilt. Paranoid veterans tend to identify primarily with other combat veterans like themselves, to treat the outside world as the enemy, and to come alive in a climate of combat. In peacetime, they often create life-and-death situations from routine occurrences. Through such unconscious processes, they are thus able to feel powerful and justify their paranoia.

Criminal Behavior

There have been attempts to correlate PTSD among Vietnam veterans with criminal behavior; the results are inconclusive because rigorous statistical analysis has not been done. Some say that Vietnam service veterans may actually be underrepresented as prison inmates in proportion to their representation in the overall population (35); others imply overrepresentation (36–38). Estimates of all incarcerated veterans have ranged from 45,000 to 125,000 at a given time with a significant percentage of these as Vietnam veterans (39).

The peak birth year of the Vietnam veteran was 1947. It is probable that no generation in American history has had greater socioeconomic expectations (40). They grew up in a period of prosperity and increasing idealism. Even the disadvantaged and minorities had hope of social betterment. The Vietnam era brought social changes and an accompanying shift in values. The harsh reality of a bitter war polarized the country, and opportunities once thought to be unlimited diminished. The optimism of the early 1960s gave way to national strife as idealism faded. Many veterans felt that they had been "chumped" (deceived) by their government and by society. The reversion to an opportunistic role during peacetime and the need to exploit others became partially a denial of their own victimization. In this way, they appeared strong rather than victimized (41). Some veterans used this as an excuse to engage in lawbreaking. In other words, I was "ripped off" . . . I will "rip off" in return.

Past moral transgressions in combat, in particular, are subject to a good deal of painful recollection, and absolution is difficult to achieve. Veterans have committed crimes with the outright motivation of getting caught (42). They are often apprehended because their mistakes are consciously or unconsciously deliberate. Getting caught and punished partially atones for the crime and partially atones for guilt for past sins. By provoking punishment, they relieve their guilt enough to be able to follow through with new offenses. The game of crime and punishment may continue interminably (43).

Drug and alcohol use and illegal activity have been long-term companions. In many instances, the use of drugs or alcohol has been a primary or ancillary factor in criminal behavior. Studies have linked PTSD and substance abuse in Vietnam veterans (44–47). The use of alcohol or drugs may have been a habit acquired in Vietnam to relieve depression and boredom, overcome undesired feelings of fear and dependence, express rebellion, or overcome inhibitions secondary to shame or guilt (41,48). If guilt persists in civilian life, the adverse consequences of drinking serve as an admirable form of self-punishment. Chronic consumption of alcohol and/or drugs may have been a coping mechanism during times of stress that later became a habit and then a contributor to criminal activity.

Some veterans may have enjoyed heightened prestige, power, and "self-realization" in Vietnam. They performed more meaningful roles (e.g., medic, squad leader) than they had been able to achieve in civilian life. As a result, some have tried to re-create the excitement they once felt by seeking altercations or by engaging in events that provide dangerous, risky, and challenging activity (e.g., flying, stunt diving, Russian roulette). Shatan (38) calls this conduct "personal duels with death." Wilson and Zigelbaum (49) says that this fulfills two unconscious aims. The behavior enhances the personal sense of being fully alive and defends against depression. It also may involve a form of repetition compulsion that serves to block the onset of intrusive experiences. He has found that these veterans only become symptomatic when blocked from physical activity. In this regard, said Wilson and Zigelbaum (49), the sensation-seeking enables the person to continue striving to master unconscious trauma by responding with self-initiated behavior that may lead to, or repeat, successful outcomes. In a psychologic sense, the veteran is compulsively repeating life-or-death encounters and mastering them with survival skills. Such sensation seeking is indiscriminate and may involve illegal activity. Wilson and Zigelbaum (49) stated that as veterans enter into sensation-seeking syndromes, they are more likely to commit nonviolent criminal acts.

Finally, during the Vietnam era, the United States military lowered standards for induction. The project designed to "rehabilitate" the poor resulted in 354,000 men entering the military who fell below the normal mental or physical requirements for entrance into the armed services (50). By lowering entry standards, the armed services dipped further into the nation's socioeconomic reservoir. It has been shown that veterans from the most unstable family backgrounds have been more likely to incur symptoms suggesting PTSD after minimal stress in Vietnam (e.g., low combat exposure or no combat) (18). Although systematic data are unavailable, some of these individuals had a criminal background and have undoubtedly contributed to veterans' postwar crime statistics.

The Duty to Protect

The above considerations are important in treating combat veterans with PTSD. In short, violence, the talk of violence, and/or preoccupation with violence is a common and inevitable aspect of treatment. Typically, the patient may express anger at the therapist, the "system," the government, or other people. When this occurs, the therapist or group leader must take a comparatively tolerant stance. In part, this strategy runs counter to prevailing forensic trends regarding the duty to protect and with psychiatry's increasing responsibility to control violence by individuals (51). The nub of the matter is the following: because exposure to violence has etiologic importance in combat-related PTSD, its verbalization in treatment can hardly be suppressed. It is not unusual for patients to make threats. When should the clinician invoke the duty to protect? The following case example epitomizes the dilemma.

Case Example

A Vietnam veteran in his 30s with several combat tours joined a veterans' therapy group. As a riverboat machine gunner in Vietnam, he had survived the sinking of several boats in combat, a short imprisonment by the enemy, and multiple gunshot wounds in battle that led to his evacuation. When his request to return to his unit was refused, he left the military. He went back to Southeast Asia as a civilian employee of another U.S. government agency where he became involved in dangerous clandestine activities. Afterward, he stayed in Southeast Asia, established a small business, and married a Thai woman with whom he had several children. He was arrested for black marketeering by a "friendly" Asian government and imprisoned for 18 months. After his release and after 6 years in Southeast Asia, he brought his family back to the United States.

When the veteran began therapy, he clearly met criteria for PTSD. He had survived many psychologically traumatic events, but two, in particular, appeared in his nightmares and haunted his waking hours: the gratuitous killing of enemy soldiers who were trying to surrender and acts of torture that he both witnessed and suffered as a prisoner. Painful as these memories were, he seemed to have an inexorable need to describe and re-create them. He often sought risk-laden adventures and would occasionally experience brief, intensely terrifying dissociative episodes when confronted with situations that resembled an aspect of earlier traumas. By self-report, he had a sporadic history of impulsive but nonlethal violence toward others and had been arrested for various civilian crimes. He claimed to own several weapons, including an automatic rifle and combat explosives that he kept as "souvenirs." He denied any use of alcohol or other disinhibiting substances.

Like many Vietnam veterans, he had a tendency to talk about violence, and frankly admitted to frequent violent fantasies. During the first group therapy session, the two therapists thoroughly discussed confidentiality limits within the group. Group members were reassured that, in most circumstances, reports of past criminal acts were confidential. Although there had been no Tarasoff-like precedent in their state, the therapists believed in their ethical duty to protect if they thought that harm to others was probable.

Several months after joining the group, the veteran expressed outrage at a utility company's "unfair" practices and threatened to "blow up" one of their remote unoccupied facilities with explosives. The therapists, observing that the patient had escalated beyond his usual stance, reiterated their obligation to take measures to protect others. He finally agreed not to act on his destructive fantasies and to contact one of the therapists instead. He denied that he would actually commit such an act but refused to agree to dispose of his explosives. He also refused voluntary hospitalization. After consulting with several supervisors and colleagues, the therapists decided that no additional actions were warranted.

In subsequent weeks, the patient twice became involved in minor, apparently impulsive acts of property destruction. He was arrested when he "tore up" a public official's office. The patient justified his actions by insisting that when the official had "interrogated" him, he had lapsed into an intrusive recollection (flashback) of his imprisonment in Southeast Asia. He was observed throwing furniture and screaming in Vietnamese. Eventually the patient was convicted of destroying public property, but because he was able to convince the court that he had experienced a combat-related flashback, he was released without significant penalty.

Nearly a year after the patient entered therapy, he arrived for a group session acting unusually quiet and looking distressed. When several group members questioned him, the patient erupted in anger. Earlier that day, he had been thwarted in his efforts to acquire an occupational license. All his rage was directed at two specific officials whom he believed were responsible. He could not be dissuaded by other group members or by the therapists from a plan to ambush the officials with an automatic firearm. Isolated in a downtown building, late in the evening, with no police or other clinicians to help, the therapists believed that they did not have the means to involuntarily hospitalize the patient. As before, he refused voluntary hospitalization and, still angry, abruptly left the clinic.

The therapists were in a quandary. On the one hand, they were well aware of the patient's penchant for rage, but they also knew that his previous violent acts had been impulsive, not calculated. It would take at least an hour for him to reach his victims. By then, maybe he would calm down; he was sober and not psychotic. On the other hand, the patient had made direct, repeated, and specific threats to kill two people. He was aware of the consequences of the action but said he no longer cared. He had suffered recent losses, including a divorce and unsuccessful child-custody battle, child-abuse allegations (later withdrawn), repeated job disappointments, arrest and conviction on a property damage charge, serious financial problems, and loss of his home. He was living in *his car and, with the exception of occasional visits from group members, had few social contacts. He recently had had difficulty controlling his angry impulses and, although there was no overt evidence of a combat fugue, he was clearly in a rage. After consulting with a supervisor by telephone, the therapists decided that immediate actions were needed to protect the potential victims from harm and the patient from ruinous consequences.*

The state police were telephoned and given information about the patient and his threats. The intended victims were also contacted and informed that there was a danger to them and that they should take measures to protect themselves.

The next day, the patient telephoned one of the therapists at work. The preceding night he had driven around for several hours before being stopped by the police. They had questioned him for some time and warned him against any attempts to harm anyone, but had taken no further action. The patient seemed initially to experience some gratification from all the attention. He denied any anger at the therapists for their actions and said that his anger at the public officials had passed. He indicated his intention to return to group the following week.

The patient, however, did not return. Instead, he sent word by another group member that he felt "betrayed" by the therapists' actions and would no longer attend the group. Several group members predicted that he would return and were proven correct when, 3 weeks later, he reappeared. When the therapists' decision to warn the potential victims was discussed, other group members reminded the patient of the therapists' intent to prevent him from doing irreparable personal damage and their earlier statements on the limits of confidentiality.

Shortly thereafter, the patient agreed to a voluntary hospitalization. Afterward, he continued in the group for another year and began weekly individual psychotherapy. Eventually he remarried, started a new family, and found employment.

Discussion

This case illustrates many common combat-related PTSD diagnostic features. The patient was well aware of his guilt and self-destructive habits, but felt helpless to curb them. The crime-and-punishment cycle was evident in the veteran's history of postwar arrests for larceny, fraud, and other property crimes. Such illegal activity may be the tip of the iceberg. It is not unusual for patients to confess past criminal activity once they have established a trusting relationship with a therapist and/or group. The crimes are usually undetected, unpunished, and distant and run the gamut from the trivial to the atrocious. Even though therapists are usually not legally obliged to report patients' past criminal acts, if crimes are particularly heinous, therapists' judgmental tolerance is strained to its limit (52). Often, the patient consciously or unconsciously expects censure from the therapist and/or other group members. It is the constancy of the therapist and the group that enables the patient to confide. For patients who express guilt, the therapist must ally himself or herself with that part of the patient's ego that now views the actions as ego-alien (53). Often patients feel they need to pay their dues or render some form of retribution before they can forgive themselves.

Describing past criminal activity is one behavior of trauma victims in therapy that evokes strong transference and countertransference feelings. Other observers have commented on the role of externalized anger when working with patients with PTSD (33, 54–57). During the first 2 or 3 months of group therapy, Vietnam veterans with PTSD characteristically ventilate their overwhelming anger toward society in general and toward the Veterans Administration (VA) Medical Center in particular, for the injustices they claim to be experiencing (57). The patients may rage at the "system" or fall back on the use of primitive combat aggression (58). Fox (59) found that 16% of his sample of 106 combat veterans manifested continuing violent behavior in civilian life. Therapists working with war survivors must have a high degree of tolerance for fantasized violence, though not for violence or for criminal activity itself. Most combat veterans appear to welcome clear limits on aggression. Such limits affirm their capacity to keep violent memories, however vivid, as memories only. The reliving of unresolved past traumatic events may then become a controlled therapeutic experience rather than a series of uncontrolled painful recollections (59).

The therapists in the case example were confronted with two separate duty to protect situations with the same patient. In the first instance, because no individuals were being threatened, they decided that the patient's commitment to call them if his violent urges intensified was sufficient. In the second instance, the patient claimed to have literally targeted two people for murder and showed no inclination to consider alternative solutions. When he abruptly left the group, the therapists had no further opportunity to influence him. If he had had a support network, a *Tarasoff* warning might not have been necessary. If there had been sufficient staff or police available, he could have been placed on a civil hold. The warning may have been unnecessary, but this is not certain. Ultimately, the patients in the group, including the patient in question, seemed to experience the action as positive.

The therapists in this case were clearly influenced by *Tarasoff* and its derivatives. The opposite influence is contained in strongly worded state statutes (60) and federal laws (61) on confidentiality. The therapists were trying to steer a course between respecting and revealing the patient's disclosures. Although the duty to protect had not been litigated in their state, they made the reasonable assumption that the court would find a *Tarasoff*-like duty if the facts fit. The Ninth Circuit Court of Appeals with federal jurisdiction in the state of Oregon has affirmed a California trial court in *Jablonski v. United States* (62) and held the government liable for a VA psychotherapist's failure to protect a veteran's common-law spouse from his dangerous propensities.

Computerized Warnings

The principle of therapeutic limit setting was applied at another level when concern about patient violence prompted the Portland, Oregon, VA Medical Center's committee on violence (Behavioral Emergency Committee [BEC]) to accept a de facto duty to warn. The medical center is a 703-bed major teaching hospital of the adjacent Oregon Health Sciences University. There are approximately 200,000 outpatient visits and 12,000 inpatient discharges per year, with significant patient clusters representing World War II and Vietnam-era veterans. The vast majority of patients are men.

The BEC was charged with the responsibility for violent-incident tracking at the medical center. The committee discovered that patients who exhibit violent behavior are often repeat performers; 25% of outpatients involved in dangerous incidents were responsible for 38% of the incidents (63). Although violent incidents represented a small percentage of ambulatory visits (approximately 0.1%), they were troublesome and dangerous. Most violent episodes involved verbal threats or conduct disturbance, but a significant percentage involved physical assault and/or weapons possession. Often, violent patients were intoxicated.

In a previous study, a sample of 48 patients who were involved in serious or repetitive violence at the Portland VA Medical Center were surveyed (63,64). The patients were all men with a mean age of 44.9 years. Violent incidents usually involved physical assault, weapon use, or both. Substance-induced organic mental disorder was the most frequent psychiatric diagnosis, followed by schizophrenia and personality disorders. Most patients also had at least one medical disorder such as a cardiovascular or gastrointestinal condition.

Although long-term prediction of dangerousness is unreliable, prediction of repeat violence by a given patient under similar circumstances may have a higher level of certainty (65). Once such high-risk patients are identified, it then becomes a question of whether it is possible to provide them with ongoing medical care without endangering other patients, visitors, or staff. Effective risk management must include identifying and setting limits on the minority of patients who are repeatedly violent. In most circumstances, violent behavior is unrecorded in charts or, when it is recorded, the warning is buried in the patient's progress notes. Frequently, staff "flag" medical records of disruptive patients with either obvious or subtle symbols; these warnings, however, may not be known to hospital house staff, who are often the most vulnerable to attack and injury.

Patients at high risk for repeat violence usually became a focus of discussion at the Portland VA BEC meetings. If there was a pattern of seriously disruptive behavior and consensus among committee members, the BEC adopted a policy of adding a recurrent computer entry, or "flag," to the patient's automated data base within the medical center–wide computer system. The flag is designed to alert medical staff to the patient's violence potential.

When a patient who has been flagged is checked in by a clerk at a computer terminal or is scheduled for an appointment, an advisory note on the computer monitor appears and a subtle audio signal is emitted. Clerks are trained to print these warnings and bring them to clinician's attention before the patient is seen. The flag includes a brief directive, such as "Patient should be searched for weapons" or "Hospital police should be asked to stand by until released by examining clinician," and usually a reference to a dated medical progress note that describes past difficulties with the patient.

The treatment team will then have the benefit of others' experience and may arrange for appropriate measures before walking into an examination room. Specific interventions may include security standby, a "show of force," and/or a search for weapons if justified by past weapons possession. If staff members have participated in hospital aggression management training, they understand the importance of a coordinated team response, the principal component of successful behavioral interventions. Perhaps more important than any specific technique is the opportunity, provided by the flag, for the staff to develop and implement a plan.

For example, one patient made 11 visits to the emergency room during a 12-month period. He often arrived in an intoxicated state after demanding that the police or ambulance driver take him to the VA hospital for treatment of injuries sustained in a street altercation. Once at the hospital, he was typically boisterous, uncooperative, and physically assaultive. In the early morning hours, when he usually appeared, he was seen by hospital house staff who were unfamiliar with his history and dependent on chart availability for information. Once an electronic flag was established, precautions could be taken, even before he arrived, to ensure treatment compliance (e.g., security officer standby, show of force by clinical staff). These measures have substantially improved his level of cooperation. Another patient had a history of threatening hospital staff. An electronic flag was added that advised security officers to stand by when the patient came to the medical center. During one visit, the patient became angry while waiting for a clinic appointment and threatened to harm a staff member. Other hospital personnel, who had been forewarned and were standing by, restrained the patient before he became assaultive.

Other methods for setting limits include confining patients to

hospital areas where they have scheduled appointments and prosecuting patients who commit violent acts (66–68). Actively involving patients' family members and friends and use of strategically
located examination or interview rooms are other practical techniques. Frequently overlooked as preventive measures are safely
designed clinic or hospital floor plans and furniture arrangements
(66,69). Preferable architectural features include patient waiting
areas that are separate from clinicians' examination rooms, two
doors in examination areas, and doors that open out; furniture
should be arranged with regard to access to the exit. At one VA
mental health clinic, staff members limited patient traffic in the
clinicians' office area by constructing a new entryway and designating a separate waiting area. The number of violent incidents at
the clinic decreased after the structural changes were made (70).

Like most medical information, precautionary flags are protected from general disclosure but are not concealed from patients.
Some patients learn about their flags by asking clerks, physicians,
or other staff members. Disgruntled patients may appeal to the
medical center's patient representative or directly to the chief of
staff under whose authority flags are instituted. The warnings do
not lessen a patient's medical evaluation or reduce benefits. On
the contrary, patients who are violence prone receive better and
more complete medical care when their behavior is under control.
The BEC has emphasized that patients are not flagged to be punished but to maintain safety and enable treatment to proceed. Each
patient flag is annually reviewed by the BEC and removed if there
is clear evidence of cooperative behavior.

So far at the Portland VA Hospital, there have been no incidents of assault on a staff member by a flagged high-risk patient.
In fact, the average number of incidents for a sample of 36 flagged
subjects declined by 91.5% during a 2.5-year study period (64).
Some of these patients had never before visited the emergency room
without physically attacking a health care worker.

Conclusion

Often, individuals with PTSD are victims of violence. Although it is not known whether patients with PTSD are more or
less violent than others, outbursts of anger are a common event in

the therapeutic setting. The therapist's decision to invoke a *Tarasoff* duty must be based on clinical circumstances. It is helpful if the therapist has a well-established relationship with the patient. Resorting to premature warnings or preventive detention may breach the patient's confidentiality and undermine trust.

Psychiatry's unwanted responsibility for violence control should not deter mental health professionals from treating violence-prone victims in an evenhanded and rational way. Concern about liability should not prevent clinicians from allowing patients to deal with their violent propensities in an open manner. There is a tendency to interpret duty to protect laws too restrictively; therefore, therapists should use reasonable care in assessing the patient's violence potential, identifying the possible victim or victims, and informing a law enforcement agency, sometimes even when no specific victim can be identified (71). In the case example, the therapist did not believe that third-party safety could be reasonably ensured by clinical interventions and, after consultation with other mental health professionals, warned that party and the relevant local law enforcement agency. Duty to protect issues are best discussed with patients before violence is threatened. In such circumstances, it has been shown that a *Tarasoff* warning or other protective actions may further the therapeutic alliance and contribute to the patient's progress in therapy (72).

Many victims of violence have a tragic view of life. Marin (73) observed that they have discovered that the world is real, the suffering of others is real, and that one's actions can sometimes irrevocably determine the destiny of others. The mistakes one makes are often transmuted directly into other's pain, and there is sometimes no way to undo that pain. For war veterans, the unacknowledged source of much anguish and anger is a deep moral distress arising from the realization that one has committed acts with real and terrible consequences and there is no way to deny one's responsibility or culpability. Mental health professionals have no easy answers for these profound moral questions, but they may be in a unique position to help certain patients diminish the cycle of violence.

References

1. Kardiner A: Traumatic neuroses of war, in American Handbook of Psychiatry, Vol 1. Edited by Arieti S. New York, Basic, 1959

2. Atkinson RM, Sparr LF, Sheff AG, et al: Diagnosis of posttraumatic stress disorder in Viet Nam veterans: preliminary findings. Am J Psychiatry 141:694–696, 1984
3. Boulanger G, Kadushin C, Rindskopf DM, et al: Posttraumatic stress disorder: a valid diagnosis? in The Vietnam Veteran Redefined: Fact and Fiction. Edited by Boulanger G, Kadushin C. Hillsdale, NJ, Lawrence Erlbaum, 1986, pp 25–35
4. Atkinson RM, Ponzoha CA, Weigel RM, et al: Assessing the validity of diagnostic criteria for posttraumatic stress disorder: a study of Vietnam veterans. Unpublished manuscript Psychiatry Service, VA Medical Center, Portland, OR
5. Lindy JD, Grace MC, Green BL: Building a conceptual bridge between civilian trauma and war trauma: preliminary psychological findings from a clinical sample of Vietnam veterans, in Post-traumatic Stress Disorder: Psychological and Biological Sequelae. Edited by Van der Kolk BA. Washington, DC, American Psychiatric Press, 1984, pp 44–57
6. Terr LG: Chowchilla revisited; the effects of psychic trauma four years after a school bus kidnapping. Am J Psychiatry 140:1543–1550, 1983
7. Fairbank JA, Keane TM, Malloy PF: Some preliminary data on the psychological characteristics of Vietnam veterans with posttraumatic stress disorders. J Consult Clin Psychol 51:912–919, 1983
8. Laufer RS, Brett E, Gallops MS: Symptom patterns associated with post-traumatic stress disorder among Vietnam veterans exposed to war trauma. Am J Psychiatry 142:1304–1311, 1985
9. Blank AS: Stresses of war: the example of Viet Nam, in Handbook of Stress. Edited by Goldberger L, Breznitz S. New York, Free Press/Macmillan, 1982, pp 631–643
10. Friedman MJ: Post-Vietnam syndrome: recognition and management. Psychosomatics 22:931–943, 1981
11. Rosenheck R: Malignant post-Vietnam stress syndrome. Am J Orthopsychiatry 55:166–176, 1985
12. Silver SM, Iacono CU: Factor analytic support for DSM-III's post-traumatic stress disorder for Vietnam veterans. J Clin Psychol 40:5–14, 1984
13. Walker JI, Cavenar JO: Vietnam veterans: their problems continue. J Nerv Ment Dis 170:174–180, 1982
14. Callen KE, Reaves ME, Maxwell MJ, et al: Vietnam veterans in the general hospital. Hosp Community Psychiatry 36:150–153, 1985
15. Foy DW, Sipprelle RC, Rueger DB, et al: Etiology of posttraumatic stress disorder in Vietnam veterans: analysis of premilitary, military

and combat exposure influences. J Consult Clin Psychol 52:79–87, 1984

16. Atkinson RM, Henderson RG, Sparr LF, et al: Assessment of Viet Nam veterans for posttraumatic stress disorder in Veterans Administration disability claims. Am J Psychiatry 139:1118–1121, 1982

17. Egendorf A, Kadushin C, Laufer RS, et al: Legacies of Vietnam: comparative adjustment of veterans and their peers, Vols 1–5 (Publ No V 101 134P-630). Washington, DC, U.S. Government Printing Office, 1981

18. Boulanger G: Predisposition to posttraumatic stress disorder, in The Vietnam Veterans Redefined: Facts and Fictions. Edited by Boulanger G, Kadushin C. Hillsdale, NJ, Lawrence Erlbaum, 1986, pp 37–50

19. Card JJ: Lives After Vietnam. Lexington, MA, Lexington Books, 1983

20. Hendin H, Pollinger A, Singer P, et al: Meanings of combat and the development of posttraumatic stress disorder. Am J Psychiatry 138:1490–1493, 1981

21. Hendin H, Pollinger A, Haas A: Combat posttraumatic stress disorders. Am J Psychiatry 141:956–959, 1984

22. Smith JR: Personal responsibility in traumatic stress reactions. Psychiatric Annals 12:1021–1030, 1982

23. Frye JS, Stockton RA: Discriminant analysis of post-traumatic stress disorder among a group of Vietnam veterans. Am J Psychiatry 139:52–56, 1982

24. Keane TM, Zimering RT, Caddall JM: A behavioral formulation of posttraumatic stress disorder in Vietnam veterans. Behav Ther 8:9–12, 1985

25. Kadushin C: Social networks, helping networks, and Viet Nam veterans, in The Trauma of War: Stress and Recovery in Viet Nam Veterans. Edited by Sonnenberg SM, Blank AS, Talbot JA. Washington, DC, American Psychiatric Press, 1985, pp 57–68

26. Keane TM, Schott WO, Chavoya GA, et al: Social support in Vietnam veterans with posttraumatic stress disorder: a comparative analysis. J Consult Clin Psychol 53:95–102, 1985

27. Archer D, Gartner R: Violent acts and violent times: a comparative approach to post war homicide rates. American Sociological Review 41:937–963, 1976

28. Shatan CF: Stress disorders among Vietnam veterans: the emotional content of combat continues, in Stress Disorders Among Vietnam Veterans. Edited by Figley CR. New York, Brunner/Mazel, 1978, pp 43–52

29. Smith C: Oral history as "therapy": combatants' accounts of the Vietnam War, in Strangers at Home. Edited by Figley CR, Leventman S. New York, Praeger, 1980

30. Fox RP: Post-combat adaptational problems. Compr Psychiatry 13:435–443, 1972

31. Eisenhart WR: You can't hack it little girl: a discussion of the covert psychological agenda of modern combat training. Journal of Social Issues 31:13–23, 1975

32. Kelman HC: Violence without moral restraint: reflections on the dehumanization of victims and victimizers. Journal of Social Issues 9:25–61, 1973

33. Egendorf A: Vietnam veterans rap groups and themes of postwar life. Journal of Social Issues 31:111–124, 1975

34. Hendin H: Combat never ends: the paranoid adaptation to post-traumatic stress. Am J Psychother 38:121–131, 1984

35. Pentland B, Rothman G: The incarcerated Vietnam-service veteran: stereotypes and realities. Journal of Correctional Education 33:10–14, 1982

36. Walker JI: Vietnam combat veterans with legal difficulties: a psychiatric problem? Am J Psychiatry 138:1384–1385, 1981

37. Doyle E, Maitland T: The Vietnam Experience: The Aftermath, 1975–85. Boston, MA, Boston Publishing, 1985

38. Shatan CF: Through the membrane of reality: "impacted grief" and perceptual dissonance in Vietnam combat veterans. Psychiatric Opinion 11:6–15, 1974

39. Brotherton GL: Post-traumatic stress disorder—opening Pandora's box? New England Law Review 17:91–117, 1982

40. Fleming RH: Post Vietnam syndrome: neurosis or sociosis? Psychiatry 48:122–139, 1985

41. Brende JO: A psychodynamic view of character pathology in combat veterans. Bull Menninger Clin 47:193–216, 1983

42. Sparr LF, Reaves ME, Atkinson RM: Military combat, posttraumatic stress disorder, and criminal behavior in Vietnam veterans. Bull Am Acad Psychiatry Law 15:141–162, 1987

43. Alexander F: Fundamentals of Psychoanalysis. New York, Norton, 1948

44. Holloway HC: Epidemiology of heroin dependency among soldiers in Vietnam. Milit Med 139:108–113, 1974

45. Sanders CR: Doper's wonderland: functional drug use by military personnel in Vietnam. Journal of Drug Issues 3:65–78, 1973

46. Robins LN: The Vietnam drug user returns (Special Action Office

Monograph, Series A, No 2). Washington, DC, U.S. Government Printing Office, 1974

47. Robins LN, Helzer JE, Davis DH: Narcotic use in Southeast Asia and afterward. Arch Gen Psychiatry 32:955–961, 1975
48. Wilson JP: Conflict, stress and growth: the effects of war on psychosocial development among Vietnam veterans, in Strangers at Home: Vietnam Veterans Since the War. Edited by Figley CR, Leventman S. New York, Praeger, 1980, pp 123–165
49. Wilson JP, Zigelbaum SD: The Vietnam veteran on trial: the relation of post-traumatic stress disorder to criminal behavior. Behavioral Sciences and the Law 1:69–83, 1983
50. Dougan C, Lipsman S: The Vietnam Experience: A Nation Divided. Boston, MA, Boston Publishing, 1984
51. Appelbaum PS: The new preventive detention: psychiatry's problematic responsibility for the control of violence. Am J Psychiatry 145:779–785, 1988
52. Appelbaum PS, Meisel A: Therapists' obligations to report their patients' criminal acts. Bull Am Acad Psychiatry Law 14:221–230, 1986
53. Haley SA: When the patient reports atrocities: specific treatment considerations of the Vietnam veteran. Arch Gen Psychiatry 30:191–196, 1974
54. Rosenheim E, Elizur A: Group therapy for traumatic neuroses. Current Psychiatric Therapies 17:143–148, 1977
55. Perconte ST: Stages of treatment in PTSD. VA Practitioner 5:47–57, 1988
56. Parson ER: Post-traumatic accelerated cohesion: its recognition and management in group treatment of Vietnam veterans. Group 9:10–23, 1985
57. Frick R, Bogart L: Transference and countertransference in group therapy with Vietnam veterans. Bull Menninger Clin 46:429–444, 1982
58. Brende JO, McCann IL: Regressive experiences in Vietnam veterans: their relationship to war, post-traumatic symptoms and recovery. Journal of Contemporary Psychotherapy 14:57–75, 1984
59. Fox RP: Narcissistic rage and the problem of combat aggression. Arch Gen Psychiatry 31:807–811, 1974
60. Oregon Revised Statutes § 40.230 Rule 504 (1986)
61. 5USC 552a Privacy Act (1974)
62. Jablonski v United States, 712 F2d 391 (9th Cir 1983)
63. Sparr LF, Drummond DJ, Hamilton NG: Managing violent patient incidents: the role of a behavioral emergency committee. QRB 14:147–153, 1988

64. Drummond DJ, Sparr LF, Gordon GH: Hospital violence reduction among high-risk patients. JAMA 261:2531–2534, 1989
65. Monahan J: Prediction research and the emergency commitment of dangerous mentally ill persons: a reconsideration. Am J Psychiatry 135:198–201, 1978
66. Soreff SM: Violence in the emergency room, in Phenomenology and Treatment of Psychiatry Emergencies. Edited by Comstock BS, Fann WE, Pokorny AD, et al. New York, Spectrum, 1984, pp 39–53
67. McCulloch LE, McNeil DE, Binder RL, et al: Effects of a weapon screening procedure in a psychiatric emergency room. Hosp Community Psychiatry 37:837–838, 1986
68. Phelan LA, Mills MJ, Ryan JA: Prosecuting psychiatric patients for assault. Hosp Community Psychiatry 36:581–582, 1985
69. Scott JR, Whitehead JJ: An administrative approach to the problem of violence. Journal of Mental Health Administration 8:36–40, 1981
70. Sparr LF, Drummond DJ: Medical center response to violent patients. Paper presented at the Oregon Psychiatric Association Fall Meeting, Ashland, OR, Sept 1986
71. Mills MJ, Sullivan G, Eth S: Protecting third parties: a decade after *Tarasoff*. Am J Psychiatry 144:68–74, 1987
72. Beck JC: When the patient threatens violence: an empirical study of clinical practice after *Tarasoff*. Bull Am Acad Psychiatry Law 10:189–201, 1982
73. Marin P: Living in moral pain. Psychology Today 6:68–74, 1981

CHAPTER ELEVEN

The Antisocial Patient

Joseph B. Layde, M.D., J.D.

Patients with antisocial personality disorder present special problems to psychiatrists, other mental health workers, and law enforcement officials. Antisocial patients may be the most likely to threaten violence. They may, in fact, have a violent past. However, they are usually what lay persons would call "sane."

When I speak of patients with antisocial personality disorder, I mean those patients who fulfill DSM-III-R (1) criteria for antisocial personality disorder. It is necessary to elicit a history of antisocial behavior beginning in childhood and persisting through adult life to make this diagnosis. Many individuals who do not fulfill the criteria for antisocial personality disorder also engage in antisocial behavior. Their diagnoses run the gamut from other personality disorders through schizophrenia and bipolar disorder. In this chapter, the terms *antisocial patient* and *sociopath* will be used as synonymous with a person fulfilling DSM-III-R criteria for antisocial personality disorder. It is important, however, to keep in mind the distinction between antisocial behavior and antisocial personality disorder.

The concept of the sociopath, or in older terminology, *psychopath*, was brilliantly outlined in all its clinical manifestations in Cleckley's *The Mask of Sanity*, first published in 1941 (2). The book has run through five revised editions, the most recent appearing in 1982 (3), and has influenced several generations of clinicians. Cleckley described individuals with antisocial personality disorder as lacking the capacity to experience true emotions. He made no claim of effective therapy for these people, but pointed out the importance of recognizing the syndrome to both the criminal justice and mental health systems.

In his 1975 article, "Sociopathy as a Human Process" (4), Vaillant maintained that sociopaths can be treated with psychotherapy, provided they were denied the ability to flee treatment. He based his contention on his experience with incarcerated patients. Cleckley and Vaillant both recognized the potential for dangerous behavior by psychopaths, but wrote little about clinical responses to that risk per se.

More recent studies of sociopathy have discussed clinical prediction of the risk of sociopaths behaving violently. In *The Menacing Stranger: A Primer on the Psychopath* (5), Grant emphasized the baffling nature of the criminal acts of psychopaths, which often do not have a clear long-term goal. The difficulty of prediction of dangerous behavior by sociopaths was examined from a legal perspective by Piperno (6), who criticized institutional psychiatrists' judgment in recommending release of offenders, including psychopaths, from indefinite commitment in a mental hospital for the criminally insane. He emphasized the well-known inability of clinicians to accurately predict future dangerous behavior over the long term. Similarly, Shapiro (7) criticized the prediction of dangerous behavior on the basis of a diagnosis of antisocial personality disorder in *Estelle v. Smith*. He pointed out that the American Psychiatric Association, in its amicus curiae brief to the U.S. Supreme Court in that case, pointed out the unreliability of psychiatric assessments of future dangerousness in the absence of information documenting a prior history of violent activities.

Very recent studies that have attempted to isolate risk factors for violence among sociopaths include the report by Heilbrun and Heilbrun (8) that dangerousness in prison and on parole among inmates of the Georgia penal system was highest among those who shared four attributes: the prisoners involved were psychopaths, had low IQs, were socially withdrawn, and had a history of prior violent crime. Sloore (9) asserted that sociopaths prone to violent behavior have a characteristic profile on the Minnesota Multiphasic Personality Inventory including elevations on scales 4 (psychopathic deviate), 6 (paranoia), 8 (schizophrenia), and 9 (hypomania). An interesting suggestion was made by Heilbrun and Gottfried (10) in a study of women in the Georgia penal system. They stated that antisociality appeared to have been a significant predictor of the dangerousness of women's criminal behavior before the rise of the women's movement in the early 1970s, but that the value of antisociality as a predictor was lost in the 1980s. They concluded that "feminism, with its emphasis on the rejection of traditional feminine values, seems to offer a new explanation of dangerous behavior in women to the extent that prior role constraints upon physical aggression are lessened" (10, p. 38).

Despite the substantial literature on the antisocial patient, there is little available that offers clinical advice on handling the issue of protecting third parties from dangerous antisocial patients.

The problem of how to protect third parties from the violence of an antisocial patient is complicated by the fact that one of the standard ways of carrying out an assumed duty to protect potential victims is to attempt civil commitment of a mentally ill patient. In many jurisdictions, the definition of mental illness required for civil commitment is something like Wisconsin's: "A substantial disorder of thought, mood, perception, orientation, or memory which grossly impairs judgment, behavior, capacity to recognize reality, or ability to meet the ordinary demands of life, but (which) does not include alcoholism" (11, p. 1065). A good argument can be made that the antisocial patient who does not suffer from a concurrent psychosis or organic condition is not "mentally ill" by such a standard.

Some court decisions assume that clinicians attempting to carry out their duty to protect endangered third parties may initiate civil commitment proceedings to detain a dangerous person. Even in those states in which physicians may initiate such an emergency detention (a list that does not include Wisconsin, where that authority is limited to law enforcement officers [12]), what is to be done when the dangerous person is antisocial but not "mentally ill" by the standard of the applicable commitment statute?

What is more, individuals with antisocial personality disorder frequently are contemptuous of authority and may go out of their way to make life difficult for clinicians, especially antisocial patients who do not initiate contact with the mental health system. Similar problems arise if antisocial patients contact the mental health system as a means of pursuing their own agenda (e.g., the procurement of controlled substances). Sociopaths often revel in authority figures' discomfiture. Sounding dangerous is frequently a device sociopaths use to get their way in the everyday world, and they may use the same tactic with the psychiatrist. Thus, clinicians may feel obliged to take some action to protect possible victims from a blustering antisocial patient, but may be hamstrung by the mental illness requirement of commitment laws and the practical difficulties of breaking patient confidentiality when there is no clear potential victim to whom the confidential information can be divulged.

On the other hand, the situation presented by the sociopath who makes an overt threat against a readily identifiable foreseeable victim is clinically different from a similar situation in which the patient making the threat suffers from, for instance, paranoid schizophrenia. For example, an antisocial man may threaten his girlfriend's life because he is jealous over her showing affection toward another man, whereas the motives behind the threat made by a man with paranoid schizophrenia might be more obscure, perhaps resulting from a persecutory delusion. In my experience, it is clinically often easier to handle the situation of such a threat in the case of the antisocial patient than in the case of a psychotic person because of the antisocial patient's good reality contact. Civil commitment may not be necessary or appropriate. The following case example illustrates such a situation. (All cases presented are composite histories.)

Case Example 1

Mr. Z is a 24-year-old black man with antisocial personality disorder who was an inpatient in a public mental health facility. He threatened the life of his girlfriend, Jane, in front of the treating psychiatrist and team nurse, saying he would shoot her after leaving the facility. The staff psychiatrist informed Mr. Z that it was important that Jane be made aware of this. Mr. Z called his girlfriend from the ward, told her of his threat, and retracted it. Mr. Z told Jane, "I was just shooting my mouth off."

A psychiatrist can often use a similar technique in clinical situations such as the one mentioned above. The technique avoids breaking confidentiality and has the advantage of enhancing communication between the parties involved in the dispute. A psychiatrist can simply inform the sociopath who has threatened a third party that there is a legal duty to somehow protect the interests of the potential victim. A psychiatrist can explain to the patient who has made the threat that it is essential that the potential victim be informed about it. The psychiatrist can then provide the patient with the opportunity to inform the victim of the threat by telephone. This often leads to a constructive communication between the sociopath and the target of the threat. The sociopath often sounds sheepish in explaining what he or she has said, and a tense situation is often defused.

A psychiatrist using this technique should insist on talking to the potential victim who has been telephoned before and after the threatener speaks, first to verify the identity of the individual on the other end of the line and after to confirm that the potential victim has received the message and to make certain that he or she feels comfortable with his or her ability to deal with the sociopath when they meet again. Given the option of speaking directly with the threatened victim or having the psychiatrist convey the threat, the sociopath will usually agree to inform the potential victim of the threat himself or herself. This affords the patient the opportunity to retract and explain the threat.

This technique is especially well suited for dealing with sociopaths, because they have the social skills to handle the telephone conversation. The technique is less likely to be of clinical assistance in the case of a paranoid schizophrenic patient who is threatening a neighbor because of a belief that the neighbor is secretly feeding nerve gas into the patient's air conditioning system. A highly delusional patient is less likely than an antisocial patient to be able to choose a societally more correct solution to the problem, such as telephoning the victim and explaining the threat.

The essential thought that should be uppermost in the clinician's mind when dealing with a potentially violent antisocial patient is how to respond clinically to the situation. The following case example illustrates some of the clinical decisions that must be made in the case of such patients.

Case Example 2

Mr. A arrived at the psychiatric crisis service (PCS), a public mental health emergency facility, at 1:15 on a winter morning with alcohol on his breath. He was accompanied by his girlfriend. Mr. A said he felt like "tearing up the place," and his girlfriend, Mary, said that Mr. A had talked just before midnight about jumping in front of a train.

A history taken at the time of his admission to the PCS revealed that Mr. A was a 28-year-old white man who had been twice married and twice divorced. He had a daughter from each of his marriages, one 10 and the other 15 years old, each living with her mother. Mr. A also had a 6-month-old son by Mary. Mr. A spoke of having some trouble with the law and said he was unemployed and not seeking work at the time.

Mental status examination performed by the resident on call at the PCS revealed Mr. A to be a young man with tattoos who looked his stated age and who was wearing a grease-smeared biker's T-shirt. He slurred his speech slightly while talking, but did not show other gross signs of alcohol intoxication. His mood was irritable, and his affect was angry. Mr. A complained that his girlfriend had "dragged him" to the hospital. Mary stated that Mr. A had talked about hurting himself earlier that night, although Mr. A said he had no intention of hurting himself. He said, however, that he intended to kill an acquaintance of his, James B, who he claimed had been making passes at Mary for several weeks.

Mr. A reported that he himself had no history of auditory or visual hallucinations, and no evidence of a formal thought disorder or of delusional thinking in his speech was found. He was oriented to person, place, and time, and his fund of general knowledge was compatible with his reported 10th-grade education. He demonstrated an adequate ability to think abstractly and to perform simple calculations. He demonstrated strikingly poor insight into the gravity of his threats to hurt himself or James B.

The resident on call summoned the staff psychiatrist and, after summarizing Mr. A's presentation, presented the question of how to respond to his threat to kill James B. The staff psychiatrist and the resident spoke to Mr. A with his girlfriend in the room. After confirming the pertinent history with Mr. A, the staff psychiatrist told him that it would be necessary to protect James B from him. The staff psychiatrist suggested that Mr. A call James and inform him of his threat, but Mary interrupted, saying, "Go ahead, call him. Tell James that I'm leaving you for him." Mr. A then refused to call James B and started to cry. He said, "I should have known.

She just wanted me around for a while to help with the kid. I'm going to go jump in front of that Amtrak train after all." Mr. A started to leave the interviewing room, but he was persuaded to sit back down. He remained adamant in his threats to kill himself.

Believing they had a duty to protect James B from Mr. A and also to protect Mr. A from committing suicide, the psychiatrists consulted with the sheriff's deputy on duty at the PCS. The deputy decided she would perform an emergency detention of Mr. A, reasoning that he was too drunk and upset to be rational, and that he was dangerous both to James B and to himself. The deputy reasoned that the determination of whether Mr. A was, in fact, mentally ill by the commitment law standards applicable would have to await his sobering up and calming down. The staff and resident psychiatrists felt that this solution clinically handled the problem, and Mr. A was admitted to the public mental health complex attached to the PCS.

Mr. A was solemn and still somewhat intoxicated at the time of his admission to a secure ward in the mental health complex. However, he went to sleep at 3:30 A.M. and slept off his intoxication. He awoke at 9:00 A.M. and began badgering nursing staff for breakfast, which he had missed while he was sleeping. He was given a sweet roll and some milk, and he began to settle down. Mr. A was still upset over the fact that he had been involuntarily detained, but he was reassured after being told by one of the nurses on the ward that a doctor would interview him later in the day to determine if it was necessary for him to be further detained against his will.

A senior psychiatric resident, who interviews patients within 24 hours of their detention by a law enforcement official, made a clinical determination about whether civil commitment proceedings should be instituted against the detainee, or whether he could be safely released, in keeping with the law in the jurisdiction involved (13).

At 2:00 P.M., the senior psychiatric resident on call interviewed Mr. A. He was no longer intoxicated and was considerably calmer. He had been closely observed by nursing staff, and there had been no indication of his attempting to harm himself or anyone else on the hospital ward. Mr. A appeared calmer during his interview with *the senior psychiatric resident than he had appeared in the PCS. He was able to give a more inclusive history than he had given in the early-morning hours.*

Mr. A had a history of pervasive antisocial conduct, starting when he was a schoolboy. He reported being truant at least once a week for a period starting in third grade. He reported that he got involved with juvenile authorities because of four shoplifting arrests when he was 12 and 13 years old. He stated that he had often started fights with his classmates as early as first grade. Mr. A related that he had been convicted twice as an adult for delivery of marijuana, that he had been convicted three times of disorderly conduct after fights when he was drinking, and that he had had his driver's license revoked after three arrests for operating a vehicle while intoxicated. Mr. A said he had worked at a series of jobs in construction, but had never held any of them for longer than a year. He said he had been unemployed three times for periods of longer than a year during which he did not seek work.

Regarding his crisis situation, Mr. A admitted his frustration over the difficulties he and his girlfriend were having in their relationship, but he reported that he felt somewhat resigned to that relationship ending soon. He pointed out that he had not felt remorse after the end of his two marriages, and he believed he would find another relationship quickly. He stated that he was very upset at James B, which concerned the senior psychiatric resident. The resident suggested again that Mr. A telephone James B and inform him of the threat. This time, Mr. A agreed. The senior psychiatric resident verified that it was James B on the telephone and listened while Mr. A explained his threat of the night before. Mr. A explained that the threat was the product of his having been drunk the night before. James B asked what would happen if Mr. A got drunk again, and Mr. A assured James that he had never had any serious thoughts of harming him, and that he believed he would have none in the future as he was reconciling himself to the end of his relationship with Mary.

The senior resident talked to James B and determined that Mr. B felt he had adequate warning and that he did not feel personally threatened by Mr. A. James B agreed to call the police if he should have any trouble with Mr. A in the future. James B assured the resident that he did not believe that his safety was in danger from Mr. A.

The senior resident discussed at some length with Mr. A the threats of harming himself and of hurting James B that he had made before admission. Mr. A attributed the threats to the situation he had been in the night before with his girlfriend and to his intoxication. He assured the resident that he was no longer thinking of suicide and that he intended to break off the relationship with his girlfriend. Mr. A reiterated his retraction of his threat to harm James B. The senior resident performed a mental status examination and determined that Mr. A had no evidence of psychosis or organic mental disease.

The senior resident thought that it was no longer possible under the law of the jurisdiction to detain Mr. A, as, in the resident's opinion, it was clear from Mr. A's mental status when not intoxicated that he did not meet the criteria for mental illness required by the commitment statute in his jurisdiction. Also, Mr. A was no longer dangerous to himself or others, in the senior resident's opinion. Accordingly, the senior resident allowed him to sign himself out of the hospital, in keeping with the above-noted provision in the commitment statute. The senior resident referred Mr. A for outpatient therapy. Before leaving the hospital ward, Mr. A telephoned his girlfriend, as he had been encouraged to do by the resident, and informed her that he would be moving out over the next few days. DSM-III-R discharge diagnoses were Axis I, alcohol intoxication (303.00); and Axis II, antisocial personality disorder (301.70) (principal diagnosis).

Mr. A attended two outpatient appointments regarding his temper. Those appointments were 1 and 2 weeks after his discharge, respectively. He stated during those sessions that he had struck up a new relationship and had moved in with another woman. He stated that he was no longer concerned with James B's overtures to his ex-girlfriend. Mr. A was not receptive to the therapist's suggestions that he enter alcohol- and drug-abuse counseling. Mr. A was lost to follow-up after his second appointment.

The history of Mr. A illustrates a number of the clinical problems that can arise in the area of confidentiality and the duty to protect in the case of a patient with antisocial personality. The clinicians involved were conversant with the laws in their jurisdiction, but they also took care to make clinically sound decisions about how to handle Mr. A during this encounter. Swartz (14) has emphasized the need for clinicians to be familiar with what he calls "local vagaries in the determination of dangerousness" (p. 67) in dealing with psychiatric emergencies. The same holds true for clinicians dealing with questions for protecting third parties.

In the case of Mr. A, the emergency room psychiatrist made an appropriate attempt to handle his threat against James B without actually breaking confidentiality: he encouraged Mr. A to call James B and tell him about the threat. Unfortunately, Mr. A was too intoxicated and upset at the time to cooperate. The emergency room clinicians were then faced with a clinical dilemma: how to handle a possibly suicidal sociopath and protect James B at the same time. They determined on a clinical basis that short-term hospitalization would be beneficial, given Mr. A's suicidality. They reasoned that, although Mr. A's espousal of dangerous ideas may have been a product of his intoxication, it was difficult for them to be sure. The legal decision was the responsibility of the sheriff's deputy. Because she was willing to sign emergency-detention papers, the first step in civil commitment proceedings, the PCS emergency room clinicians felt that they were able to protect James B and to protect Mr. A from himself pending clarification of the clinical issues. They made their clinical decision to admit Mr. A in the context of the legal determination by the deputy that emergency detention was permissible.

The senior resident who saw Mr. A the next day made his clinical decisions on the basis of good knowledge of the laws of his jurisdiction and through the application of his clinical judgment and common sense. The successful suggestion to Mr. A that he telephone James B and discuss the threat with him handled the clinical problem of Mr. A's behavior and the legal problem of the possible duty to protect James B without actually violating confidentiality.

A clinician facing a patient who was unwilling to make that telephone call might have had to violate confidentiality and inform James B and law enforcement officials of Mr. A's threat. However, the senior resident on call used his skills as an empathic communicator to lead Mr. A to see that making the telephone call was the best solution to both the clinical and legal problems. Carlson et al. (15) emphasized the fact that in cases of threats to third parties by a patient, "involvement of the patient is extremely important and serves the purpose of limit setting for which the patient may be grateful" (p. 184). In the case of Mr. A, an antisocial patient, limit setting was particularly important. One cannot always expect that an antisocial patient will be grateful for such actions, however.

The following case example illustrates that the solution of legal problems with antisocial patients can be quite problematic.

Case Example 3

Mr. W is a 29-year-old white man who arrived in the PCS at 9:30 P.M. on a December evening accompanied by two police officers. One of the officers stated that he had seen Mr. W kicking his motorcycle furiously after it had slid out from under him in the fresh snow. According to the officer, Mr. W did not appear intoxicated, but looked so angry and bent on destroying his motorcycle that the officer called for his partner. The two police officers approached Mr. W and told him they thought he should be evaluated at the PCS. The officers gave him the alternative of accompanying them to the PCS or being arrested for disorderly conduct. He angrily accompanied them.

After the officers delivered Mr. W to the PCS and left, the psychiatric resident on call asked Mr. W what was troubling him. He shouted at the resident, "That damn motorcycle mechanic, Tom, really screwed me over again. He sold me some lousy retread tires, and I nearly killed myself when I wiped out in the snow. That's the third time Tom's messed with my bike. I'm going to go get my shotgun and blow a hole in that rinky-dink shop he works in!" The resident tried to calm Mr. W down by asking him some background questions, but Mr. W remained furious. The resident did not notice any alcohol on Mr. W's breath. Mr. W was dressed appropriately for the cold in a black leather jacket. When the resident could not engage him in conversation about anything other than his anger over his motorcycle mishap, the resident asked Mr. W for more information about the mechanic and garage he had threatened. Mr. W became quite agitated and said to the resident, "I'm not telling you nothing. You're just trying to mess with me, just like those cops." With that, Mr. W suddenly jumped up from his chair in the PCS examination room and bolted out an open door into the winter chill.

The psychiatric resident spoke to the staff psychiatrist and told him of Mr. W's threat. There were over 200 garages in the city, and, the clinicians guessed, many of them had a mechanic named Tom. The staff psychiatrist recommended to the resident that they call the police and tell them the little they knew of Mr. W's threat, although they realized that it was difficult to foresee who might be the victim of any possible violence coming from Mr. W, given the paucity of available information.

The most important point illustrated in the case examples described is that clinical decision making should guide psychiatrists in various jurisdictions in their attempts to reconcile local law, with which they must be familiar, with the best interests of the patient and any potential victims of the patient. The question of whether to violate confidentiality can often, but not always, be finessed. In some situations, the clinician may find that he or she must violate confidentiality and warn the potential victim of a sociopath of impending danger. The decision to hospitalize, like the other questions faced by the clinicians who dealt with Mr. A, the intoxicated, suicidal sociopath in the second case example, was handled in a clinically appropriate way. In other circumstances, or in other jurisdictions, it might have been appropriate to handle Mr. A differently. The psychiatrists involved did not have to make the determination of whether Mr. A was, in fact, "mentally ill" at the time of his emergency detention, because the deputy sheriff made the determination to detain him. No matter where or how a psychiatrist is presented with the problem of a potentially dangerous antisocial patient, clinical judgment, informed by a knowledge of the law in the psychiatrist's jurisdiction, should be the basis of decision making.

Psychiatrists and other mental health professionals often feel so encumbered by their possible legal liability when dealing with a potentially dangerous antisocial patient that they lose the ability to think clearly and to rely on their clinical judgment. This need not be the case. No one can guarantee that a psychiatrist will never be sued by a third party injured by a patient. Nevertheless, good clinical judgment is still the best guide for the clinician in practice, especially in dealing with a potentially dangerous patient, particularly one with antisocial personality disorder.

References

1. American Psychiatric Association: Diagnostic and Statistical Manual of Mental Disorders, 3rd Edition, Revised. Washington, DC, American Psychiatric Association, 1987, pp 344–346
2. Cleckley HM: The Mask of Sanity. St. Louis, MO, CV Mosby, 1941
3. Cleckley HM: The Mask of Sanity, Revised. New York, New American Library, 1982
4. Vaillant GE: Sociopathy as a human process. Arch Gen Psychiatry 32:178–183, 1975
5. Grant VW: The Menacing Stranger: A Primer on the Psychopath. Oceanside, NY, Dabor, 1977
6. Piperno A: Indefinite commitment in a mental hospital for the criminally insane: two models of administration of mental health. Journal of Criminal Law and Criminology 65:520–527, 1974
7. Shapiro DL: Constitutional issues in forensic psychiatry: *Estelle v. Smith*, the "government doctors," legal constraints on psychological examinations. American Journal of Forensic Psychology 2:55–59, 1984
8. Heilbrun AB, Heilbrun MR: Psychopathy and dangerousness: comparison, integration and extension of two psychopathic typologies. Br J Clin Psychol 24:181–195, 1985
9. Sloore H: Use of the MMPI in the prediction of dangerous behavior. Acta Psychiatr Belg 88:42–51, 1988
10. Heilbrun AB, Gottfried DM: Antisociality and dangerousness in women before and after the women's movement. Psychol Rep 62:37–38, 1988
11. Wisconsin Statutes § 51.01 (13) (b), 1988
12. Wisconsin Statutes § 51.15 (4–5), 1988
13. Wisconsin Statutes § 51.15 (5), 1988
14. Swartz MS: What constitutes a psychiatric emergency: clinical and legal dimensions. Bull Am Acad Psychiatry Law 15:57–68, 1987, p 67
15. Carlson RJ, Friedman LC, Riggert SC: The duty to warn/protect: issues in clinical practice. Bull Am Acad Psychiatry Law 15:179–186, 1987

CHAPTER TWELVE

Driving, Mental Illness, and the Duty to Protect

Sally L. Godard, M.D.
Joseph D. Bloom, M.D.

The physician's duty to protect third parties from the violent actions of patients has evolved in the 15 years since the *Tarasoff* decisions of the California Supreme Court. *Tarasoff*-like cases have emerged in many jurisdictions, with this duty frequently expanded to include protection from actions against unidentified third parties and property (1–4).

The past decade has also witnessed greater public attention to driving and its potential harms. Awareness of the motor vehicle as a dangerous weapon, especially when combined with alcohol use, has increased. Organizations such as Mothers Against Drunk Driving (MADD) have been successful in educating the public and in securing legislation that relates to driving and alcohol use. Heightened public opinion and tighter laws and regulations have influenced the actions of juries and judges.

This continued judicial focus on both the duty to protect and the motor vehicle as a potentially lethal weapon created a situation that was just waiting to happen. It was only a matter of time before cases involving the mentally ill driver would emerge.

Courts have been confronted with cases alleging that physicians are liable for injuries in motor vehicle accidents involving their patients who drive. These cases can be divided into four categories. Many have been considered to be malpractice cases based on the physician's failure to warn the patient that a prescribed medication may impair driving ability (5). Other cases have been based on state statutes that require a reporting by physicians of patients with conditions that may affect their ability to drive (5).

A third type of case, modeled on the *Tarasoff* decisions, speaks to an obligation to protect the public that is not based on statute (1,3). In a fourth category, the liability of the physician is premised on other statutes that may involve a responsibility to protect society (6,7).

Cain v. Rijken (6,7) represents this fourth category of case law. Although not a *Tarasoff*-type case, it has been handled as such by the state and, as a result, has influenced the practice of psychiatry in the state of Oregon. In this chapter we explore the historical framework related to driving and mental illness that existed in Oregon before *Cain v. Rijken*. We will then describe the case in more detail and highlight the administrative changes resulting from this important case. The clinical dilemma faced by psychiatrists who are involved with mentally ill drivers in the community and state hospitals will be emphasized with two case examples that represent a composite of our experience. We conclude with a discussion of the major issues and our recommendations for the role of psychiatrists.

Statutory Background

Several Oregon statutes are pertinent to the issues of driving and mental illness. Statutes governing the activities of the Oregon Motor Vehicles Division outline the eligibility rules for driving. A motor vehicle code statute (8) originating in the early 1930s defines those not eligible for driving privileges and includes persons civilly committed to a mental institution:

(5) A person declared not eligible to be issued a license under this subsection may become eligible by establishing to the satisfaction of the division that the person is competent to operate a motor vehicle safely with respect to persons and property and:
(a) The person has been declared competent by judicial decree;
(b) The person has been released from the state institution upon a certificate of the superintendent of the institution that the person is competent; or
(c) The person has established eligibility in accordance with ORS 807.090

In addition to those civilly committed, the state defines other categories of individuals who may be ineligible to drive:

(6) A person the [Motor Vehicles] division reasonably believes is afflicted with or subject to any condition which brings about momentary or prolonged lapses of consciousness or control that is or may become chronic.

(7) A person the division reasonably believes is suffering from a physical or mental disability or disease serving to prevent the person from exercising reasonable and ordinary control over a motor vehicle while operating it upon the highways.

It is important to note the reference to competency in Section 5 of the above statute. This older statute assumes an incompetence of committed state hospital patients that is in contradiction with a mental health statute from the 1960s that declares that "no person admitted to a state hospital for the treatment of mental illness shall be considered by virtue of the admission to be incompetent" (9). Statutes also outline the method of establishing eligibility for those with disease or disability that may otherwise render them ineligible (10). This procedure involves obtaining a certificate of eligibility from the Health Division. To meet the qualifications for a certificate may require a report from the applicant's physician or a physician designated by the Health Division. The Motor Vehicle Code goes on to require reporting of

All persons authorized by the state of Oregon to diagnose and treat disorders of the nervous system shall report immediately to the Health Division every person over 14 years of age diagnosed as having a disorder characterized by momentary or prolonged lapses of consciousness or control that is, or may become, chronic. (11)

Cain v. Rijken

In *Cain v. Rijken*, a wrongful death claim was brought by the personal representative of an individual who was killed in an automobile accident by the defendant, Paul Rijken. At the time of the accident in 1981, Mr. Rijken was under the jurisdiction of the Oregon Psychiatric Security Review Board (PSRB) (12) after being found not guilty by reason of insanity for a previous crime. After a period of hospitalization, the PSRB placed Mr. Rijken on monitored conditional release in a day treatment program in a community hospital. At one point during the conditional release, Mr. Rijken began to experience increased symptoms of his mental illness. The program attempted to treat this problem with hospitalization in the community and closer monitoring of his behavior. Unfortunately, during this time, Mr. Rijken operated a motor vehicle in a reckless manner. While speeding through an intersection, he caused the accident that resulted in the death of two persons, one who was represented in this suit.

The trial court granted a summary judgment in favor of the day treatment program. When the plaintiff appealed, the court of appeals reversed the summary judgment and remanded the case for trial. This decision focused on whether the treatment program was obligated by a duty to protect the deceased individual. The appellate court based its ruling on PSRB statutes, which delineate the duty of the review board: "In determining whether a person should be committed to a state hospital, conditionally released or discharged, the board shall have as its primary concern the protection of society" (13). The statutes emphasize that the PSRB jurisdiction over a person continues until that person "no longer presents a substantial danger to others" (14). The opinion stated that the treatment program was, therefore, responsible to exercise reasonable care to control the "dangerous propensities of the patient" and whether the program failed to meet this obligation was a matter for a trial court to determine.

The Oregon Supreme Court upheld the court of appeal's reversal, stating that a breach of the duty of reasonable care in treating patients and controlling their acts creates potential liability to persons who are foreseeably endangered. The court held that a jury should determine if the risk to members of the public not specifically identifiable was foreseeable in this case. The case was, thereafter, remanded to the trial court. The parties settled out of the courtroom, and the case was closed.

Although the court stated that its decision was based on PSRB statutes and not on the *Tarasoff* doctrine, we believe that state government responded as if this were a *Tarasoff* case. This decision has also become part of the case law that has evolved across the country following the *Tarasoff* decision (15).

Administrative Policy Changes Since *Cain v. Rijken*

Cain v. Rijken strongly influenced opinion in both the Motor Vehicles Division and the Mental Health Division. This led to policy changes in both arenas that affected the lives of patients and the practice of clinicians.

Motor Vehicles Division Response

An initial response by the Motor Vehicles Division to *Cain v. Rijken* was the initiation of two statutory changes. One required mandatory reporting of any person under PSRB jurisdiction who was involved in a traffic violation or accident (16). The second established that the superintendent of a state psychiatric hospital be required to notify the Motor Vehicles Division of any discharged person who, in the opinion of the superintendent, should not drive because of his or her mental condition (17). Another response resulted when the circuit court judge who presided over a trial of a lawsuit brought by the parents of the second man killed addressed the administrators of the Motor Vehicles Division with a message from the jury. The jury criticized the Motor Vehicles Division for not meeting a statutory obligation:

> We do believe . . . that the application form used by the Division of Motor Vehicles to obtain or reinstate an Oregon Driver's License does not fulfill their responsibility to comply with the statute stating that the [Division of] Motor Vehicles must screen for physical and *mental* impairment. (18)

At that time, the standard forms questioned applicants about physical impairments that may affect the ability to drive (e.g., epilepsy, stroke, or diabetes) but did not screen for history of mental impairment.

As a result of the judge's and jury's action, the Motor Vehicles Division in April 1987 amended its forms to include a broad screening for mental impairment. The question on the initial and renewal application forms asks if the applicant has or has been treated for a mental disorder in the past 4 years. If the applicant answers in the affirmative, he or she would then be required to obtain a "Driver Medical Certification" signed by the treating physician. This certification obligates the doctor to provide diagnostic and medication information along with findings from the history or physical examination. The physician then is required to answer whether "this patient is medically qualified to safely operate a motor vehicle." The following case example illustrates this procedure.

Case Example 1

Mr. K is a 27-year-old single man with an 8-year history of schizophrenia. He has been hospitalized three times, the last hospitalization occurring 2 years ago. Although he has lived independently in the past, he currently lives with his parents in a suburban community. His schizophrenic symptoms are under fair control with his neuroleptic medication. He no longer hears voices except under stressful conditions. He maintains some paranoid feelings but has no fixed delusional system.

Mr. K receives services from a local mental health program. He sees a psychiatrist monthly and meets with his case manager each week. He has been involved in day treatment since his last hospitalization. Because of his gradual improvement, his treatment plan was recently changed and he began a vocational rehabilitation program that would lead to supported work activities. Although he and his treatment team continue to struggle with his negative symptoms of schizophrenia, Mr. K's insight into his illness and his active interest in treatment have decreased his disabilities.

Mr. K received the standard renewal form for a driver's license in the mail. He sent in the proper information, including the information that he is diagnosed with a mental illness. When the letter arrived from the Motor Vehicles Division requiring that he receive a letter of certification from his physician concerning his ability to drive, Mr. K became worried. Would he lose his license? If he did, how could he continue the activities in which he was involved? He presented the letter to his case manager, who forwarded it to the *psychiatrist. Added to the questions of Mr. K are the questions of the psychiatrist. Can this patient drive? On what criteria can I make a recommendation? What will be the consequences of my recommendation?*

With the response of the Motor Vehicles Division, psychiatrists in the community and private sector are faced with new diagnostic challenges of their patients' driving ability, and the state psychiatric hospitals now have a clear duty to identify impaired drivers.

Mental Health Division Response

In the state psychiatric hospitals, psychiatrists became responsible for reporting to the superintendent any discharged patients who are potentially incapable of driving. To assist in this identification, the state hospitals revised their medical record procedures in 1986 to provide guidelines for physicians making this determination. Patients who were to be strongly considered as impaired included

1. Individuals who cannot read or interpret road signs as a result of mental illness.
2. Individuals with loss of judgment, concentration, or motor control resulting from symptoms of mental disorder. (Hallucinations, delusions, severe anxiety, agitation, panic elation, hyperactivity with careless or reckless behaviors, and explosive anger episodes with aggressive behavior dangerous to others strongly suggest impairment.)
3. Individuals subject to loss of alertness or motor control secondary to side effects of psychotropic medication. (Dizziness, dystonia, rigidity, bradykinesia, akathisia, drowsiness, or sedation should be carefully considered.)
4. Individuals having a history of poor compliance with treatment resulting in recurrent psychotic episodes during which a lack of control would result in hazardous operation of a motor vehicle.
5. Individuals with specific delusions or hallucinations related to driving a motor vehicle that would result in substantial loss of ability to control a motor vehicle.

It is noteworthy that the number of driver's license suspensions resulting from notification by the state hospital increased from 99 in 1985 to 352 in 1986 and 375 in 1987 as a consequence of the *Cain v. Rijken* furor.

Case Example 2

Ms. S is a college-educated, 33-year-old woman hospitalized for the fourth time in 5 years at an Oregon state hospital. The most recent admission in July, in which she was civilly committed and placed in the state hospital, lasted more than 3 months.

Ms. S has bipolar illness and is usually hospitalized during a manic episode. Before her commitment, she had been living alone in her apartment. She stopped taking her medications several months earlier. During mid-June, Ms. S gradually began to feel as if she had more energy. She stayed up most of the night, working on her household and gardening chores. Along with her increased energy, she also became more irritable and demanding. Her neighbors complained of her loud behavior, but backed off when she responded with angry accusations. Finally, one evening, she was apprehended by the police. They had been notified that a woman in a long flowing robe was flagging down cars from the middle of a busy intersection. Ms. S was placed on a peace officer's hold in a community hospital and, thereafter, was committed and transferred to the state hospital.

During her hospitalization, Ms. S began taking an antipsychotic and lithium once again. Her manic episode subsided substantially after about 2 weeks, and she continued to improve throughout her hospital stay. At the time of discharge, she was thinking clearly with appropriate affect. No evidence of grandiose or delusional ideation persisted. Arrangements were made for her to stay with a relative until she was able to live independently again. She was scheduled to be seen by a case manager at the county mental health clinic the following week.

The hospital physician faced the task of determining the patient's ability to drive. This example raises more questions than answers. What was this woman's previous driving ability? Could her current mental status interfere with her ability to drive? How do her medications affect her driving? What is the likelihood that she may discontinue treatment, and will this affect her driving ability? The physician struggles with the questions.

Literature Review

In examining the administrative changes that occurred as a result of *Cain v. Rijken* and considering the effects for both patients and clinicians, a nagging question remains. Although statutory law and administrative policy are based on an assumption of the poor driving ability of the mentally ill, is this assumption valid? The empirical evidence is limited and inconclusive.

In an early Canadian study, Tillman and Hobbs (19) investigated the personality characteristics and social background of nearly 100 drivers with a record of four or more accidents. They found that accident-prone drivers are more aggressive and impulsive with histories that include delinquency, family disruption, and unstable employment. This provided early empirical data to support an "accident-prone" personality.

When Waller (20) considered the driving records of persons in California with chronic mental conditions known to the Department of Motor Vehicles, he found that persons with mental illness (defined as primarily schizophrenia and bipolar illness) had accident rates twice that of the comparison group.

Crancer and Quiring (21) found a higher accident rate for persons with personality disorders and neurosis but a rate comparable to the comparison group for persons with schizophrenia. Selzer (22) studied fatal accidents in Michigan. The fatality group showed more paranoid ideation, clinical depression, and suicidal proclivity than did the control group. Eelkema et al. (23) confirmed that persons with personality disorders have higher accident rates but found that persons with psychosis had higher accident rates before hospitalization but lower rates after discharge. Despite general agreement that persons with antisocial personality disorders and alcoholism have an increased risk of motor vehicle accidents (24), Tsuang et al. (25), in a comprehensive review, stated the need for empirical studies with more rigorous designs and more subjects that would test hypotheses regarding the role of the major mental illnesses and driving ability.

When the American Medical Association (AMA) published its opinion on medical conditions affecting drivers (26), the extreme difficulty of assessing driving impairments caused by psychiatric disorders was recognized. They did note that some psychiatric conditions may impair an individual's ability to drive, highlighting schizophrenic disorders, paranoid disorders, affective disorders, and disorders of alcohol use. The AMA did assign responsibility to the physician by stating, "Prevention of motor vehicle crashes depends upon the physician's recognition of persons in these high risk groups and upon skillful assessments made during the times of their greatest vulnerability" (p. 36).

Discussion

The legal decision in *Cain v. Rijken* was a narrow elaboration of the law in Oregon governing insanity acquittees under the PSRB. It was based on a statute that clearly specifies public safety as a number one priority. It appears to us that the subsequent policy changes went far beyond the courts and provide us with an interesting example of an administrative agency expansion of *Tarasoff* in Oregon. The broadened interpretation of the duty to protect by the Mental Health Division and the Motor Vehicles Division clearly affects the lives of persons with mental illness and the clinical practice of psychiatrists in Oregon.

The initial revision of the application and renewal licensing forms of the Motor Vehicles Division screened broadly for a mental disorder with the initial assumption that persons with mental illness may be at risk to drive. In addition, there was the assumption in the Motor Vehicles Code (8) that originated in the 1930s that all persons in the state hospital were incompetent and thus unable to drive. This was probably a widely held view at the time. However, in the past two decades, civil commitment laws have been modified, and commitment is no longer synonymous with incompetence (9). Therefore, it is apparent that the initial response of the Motor Vehicles Division was based on an outdated view of mental illness and incompetence. This response required that a large number of individuals prove that they were able to drive, rather than the Motor Vehicles Division identifying the persons who were not able to drive.

The Mental Health Division responded to the situation by attempting to establish criteria for reporting hospitalized patients to the Motor Vehicles Division based on an assumed association between symptoms and driving. With these criteria, the hospital greatly increased the number of cases reported to the Motor Vehicles Division from 99 in 1985 to an average of 364 in 1986 and 1987. The accuracy of these reports and their consequences for patient adjustment have not been assessed. If this increased reporting represents an overreaction to liability concerns, then it may be at the expense of our patients.

Another issue for patients with mental illness is that the process for obtaining verification of "competency" requires that individuals allow their psychiatric history and records to be submitted to the Motor Vehicles Division. Although this information is said to be confidential within the division, when public interest is considered to outweigh the value of confidentiality, these records may become accessible in the future.

The consequences for the practicing psychiatrist are equally unfortunate. First, it is important to reflect on how these decisions affect the standard of treatment in the psychiatric community. Whereas it has always been the physician's responsibility to discuss the side effects of medications, including those that may affect driving ability, it has not been the physician's duty to make sure that the patient does not drive. Nor has it been standard practice for physicians to routinely inquire about a patient's driving ability. Few psychiatrists have ever witnessed their patients' driving, and their knowledge of a patient's driving ability is limited. This is well illustrated by the first case example in which the psychiatrist struggled to complete the form that would determine whether Mr. K would get his license. The psychiatrist was being asked to offer an opinion on an issue that previously had not been within the domain of the physician's duty.

The second difficulty facing the clinician involves the ability to predict dangerousness. It is well established that psychiatrists and other mental health professionals are not able to predict long-term dangerousness (27). The psychiatric profession agrees that such predictions should not be made in forensic settings. These predictions are also not valid in hospital or clinic practices.

In the second case example, the hospital physician stated in the discharge summary that Ms. S was not capable of driving due to a history of erratic driving. The hospital obtained information in her driving record from the Motor Vehicles Division. It showed that she had six previous violations, five for speeding and one for improper registration stickers. Note that the treating physician's decision was based in large measure on her driving record. Though the decision may have been appropriate, because past behavior is one of the best predictors of future behavior, this driving history was not the exclusive knowledge of the physician but, rather, originated from the source to which the recommendation was made. Therefore, the decision could not be considered to be clinically based but did serve to protect the hospital from future claims of discharging a potentially dangerous driver.

Presented with these prominent issues for people with mental illness and psychiatrists in practice, we offer the following recommendations for clinicians and policymakers.

First, although psychiatrists have a duty to address the issue of driving and safety with their patients as it relates to the symptoms of mental illness and the possible side effects of medications, they should actively resist any attempt from others to have them shoulder the responsibility for the prediction of driving ability. It is not the duty of the psychiatrist to screen for and protect society from a potentially disabled driver. This responsibility lies with the Motor Vehicles Division, which maintains the driving records and has the ability to test the individual driver.

Oregon's psychiatrists and state employees have begun to address this issue. Since the modification of license application and renewal forms in April 1987 that resulted in requiring persons with a mental illness to obtain a report from their physician affirming or denying their ability to drive, psychiatrists have opposed this procedure on the basis of their inability to predict. This confrontation led to a work group consisting of Motor Vehicles Division and Mental Health Division staff with representatives from other organizations, including the American Civil Liberties Union and the Oregon Psychiatric Association. A revision is now in progress that requires the applicant to state whether a mental illness has ever interfered with his or her ability to drive. If the applicant answers in the affirmative, the physician is asked to submit clinical information, but not a recommendation on the patient's driving ability or a prediction of potential dangerousness.

Second, the mental health community has an obligation to support the patient's desire for confidentiality. It is because of this privilege of confidentiality that many people are willing to seek mental health treatment. If citizens are discouraged from obtaining treatment because of a fear that this may become more widely known, then neither the state nor the individual benefits.

Third, further empirical research should be undertaken. If we wish to assess the driving ability of persons in certain diagnostic categories, the studies must not be limited to individuals in a hospital setting. Large samples that are compared with control groups with the same demographic characteristics are essential. Certainly, the factor of substance abuse in the mentally ill patient and its consequences for driving must not be overlooked as we correlate traffic violations and accidents with mental illness.

These recommendations represent a beginning as we examine the complicated issues of mental illness and driving. As we gather the data that may provide us with some answers, mental health professionals must constantly be aware of the assumptions and ramifications that result from public policy decisions. This chapter illustrates how far the administrative expansion of a narrow court decision can reach into the lives of mentally ill persons and those who treat them.

References

1. Petersen v Washington, 671 P2d 230, 100 (Wash 421 1983)
2. Stone AA: Vermont adopts *Tarasoff*: a real barn-burner. Am J Psychiatry 143:352–355, 1986
3. Naidu v Laird, 539 A2d 1064 (Del Sup Ct 1988)
4. Bloom JD, Rogers JL: The duty to protect others from your patients—*Tarasoff* spreads to the northwest. West J Med 148:231–234, 1988
5. Sarno G: Liability of physician, for injury to or death of third party, due to failure to disclose driving-related impediment. 43 Annotated Law Review 4th, p 153–171
6. Cain v Rijken, 717 P2d 140, 300 (Ore 706 1986)

7. Cain v Rijken, 700 P2d 1061, 74 (Ore App 76 1985)
8. Oregon Revised Statute 807.060 (subsection 5,6,7)
9. Oregon Revised Statute 426.295 (subsection 1)
10. Oregon Revised Statute 807.090
11. Oregon Revised Statute 807.710 (subsection 1)
12. Rogers JL, Bloom JD: The insanity sentence: Oregon's psychiatric security review board. Behavioral Sciences and the Law 3:69–84, 1985
13. Oregon Revised Statute 161.336 (subsection 10)
14. Oregon Revised Statute 161.351 (subsection 1)
15. Beck JC (ed): The Potentially Violent Patient and the *Tarasoff* Decision in Psychiatric Practice. Washington, DC, American Psychiatric Press, 1985
16. Oregon Revised Statute 807.410
17. Oregon Revised Statute 807.700
18. Snouffer WC: Letter to Oregon Motor Vehicles Division, Attachment A. March 27, 1985
19. Tillman WA, Hobbs GE: The accident prone automobile driver. Am J Psychiatry 106:321–331, 1949
20. Waller JA: Chronic medical conditions and traffic safety. N Engl J Med 273:1413–1420, 1965
21. Crancer A, Quiring DL: The mentally ill as motor vehicle operators. Am J Psychiatry 126:807–813, 1969
22. Selzer ML: Alcoholism, mental illness, and stress in 96 drivers causing fatal accidents. Behav Sci 14:1–10, 1969
23. Eelkema RC, Brosseau J, Koshnick R, et al: A statistical study on the relationship between mental illness and traffic accidents—a pilot study. Am J Public Health 60:459–469, 1970
24. Noyes R: Motor vehicle accidents related to psychiatric impairment. Psychosomatics 26:569–580, 1985
25. Tsuang MT, Boor M, Fleming JA: Psychiatric aspects of traffic accidents. Am J Psychiatry 142:538–546, 1985
26. Doege TC, Engelberg AL (eds): Medical Conditions Affecting Drivers. American Medical Association, 1986, pp 7–9, pp 36–40
27. Monahan J: The clinical prediction of violent behavior. Washington, DC, U.S. Government Printing Office, 1981

CHAPTER THIRTEEN

The Case of Ms. Troubled

M s. Troubled was in her mid-20s when she began psychotherapy with Dr. Senior, an experienced psychiatrist. She complained of severe feelings of anxiety, at times bordering on panic. She also experienced episodes of depression and hopelessness lasting anywhere from several hours to several weeks. She reported great difficulty in maintaining herself affectively on an even keel.

She had been briefly but intensely involved with several men. In each case, she had quickly become attached and several times had sexual relations with men she barely knew. Typically, the men would disappoint her and she would break up with them, often after vicious arguments or fights. In at least one case, she was a victim of date rape after she went home with a man she met in a bar.

Ms. Troubled reported that at times she had feelings of unreality, as if she were separated from other people by an invisible barrier. She had superficially slashed her wrists on several occasions in an effort to "feel something." She had a history of drinking, at times to the point of oblivion. She had used marijuana as a teenager, but had stopped after one frightening episode of paranoia.

She had completed high school and 1 year of business college. Her secretarial skills were excellent, but she had lost several jobs, either quitting abruptly when she felt her boss had let her down, or precipitating arguments that led to her being asked to leave.

Her parents had separated when she was 5 and divorced when she was 7. Her mother remarried when the patient was 8. Beginning when she was 10, her stepfather began to abuse her sexually. He repeatedly performed cunnilingus on her, and when she was ages 13–15 they had sexual intercourse. On several occasions, she tried to tell her mother, but her mother changed the subject and shooed her out of the room. At age 15, she ran away from home, was brought back, and precipitated a family crisis by insisting that she would not stay in the same house with her stepfather. Extended family members agreed to take her in. She lived with them until she was 18 and had been on her own ever since.

Ms. Troubled was quite bright and psychologically minded, and she had excellent health insurance. Dr. Senior treated her in intensive individual psychotherapy twice a week for several years. He also prescribed antidepressants and low doses of antipsychotics.

Initially, she was guarded, shy, and frightened. Slowly, she began to trust Dr. Senior. She also began to be interested in him personally. They lived in a small community, and facts about him were readily available.

Ms. Troubled gradually formed an intense, idealized transference, and began to express feelings of hostility toward Dr. Senior's wife and jealousy of his children. She told Dr. Senior of her fantasies of killing his wife or children, perhaps by putting a poisonous snake in his wife's car.

Dr. Senior did not believe the patient intended to act on these threats, and he dealt with them as a therapeutic issue, making transference interpretations. He linked these fantasies to her wishes for the idealized absent father, her rage at her mother who had failed to protect her from her stepfather, and her intense ambivalence toward her stepfather as well as her guilt about her sexual involvement with him.

The transference grew increasingly difficult to handle. The patient began to express erotic fantasies about the psychiatrist, and fantasies about becoming part of his family. Ultimately, Dr. Senior became convinced that this therapy was not constructive. The interpretation of the fantasies had not served to diminish their intensity. After obtaining consultation with four experienced colleagues, Dr. Senior decided it would be best if he and Ms. Troubled terminated, and over a period of several months, they did terminate the therapy. Dr. Senior gave his patient the names of several other therapists who would potentially be available to see her.

Shortly after termination, Ms. Troubled began simultaneously to see two new mental health professionals for evaluation. She told neither that she was seeing the other.

She went to a pet store and asked to purchase a poisonous snake. The owner asked whether she knew how to handle it, and when she assured him she did, he sold it to her. She put the snake in a box that she wrapped as a package, and she addressed the package to Dr. Victim, whose office was next door to Dr. Senior's. She then left the package with the office receptionist.

Ms. Troubled immediately went home and telephoned both of her new therapists, telling each of them that she had arranged for a poisonous snake to be delivered to Dr. Victim. Neither therapist acted on this information immediately. After 48 hours, one called Dr. Victim's office to report this conversation. The same receptionist who had accepted the package from Ms. Troubled took this call. Fortunately, Dr. Victim had been away, so the package was still in her mailbox. The receptionist retrieved it.

The receptionist then informed Dr. Victim and the authorities that there was possibly a poisonous snake in her mailbox. The authorities came and removed the package. Ultimately they ascertained that the snake was poisonous. The package also contained an unsigned note threatening to kill Dr. Victim. When the receptionist learned this, she informed Dr. Victim that Ms. Troubled had delivered the package.

Dr. Victim was terrified. She had no relationship with the patient and initially no idea why this had happened. Conversation with the receptionist clarified that the woman who left the package was a former patient of Dr. Senior. Dr. Victim learned from Dr. Senior that the patient had threatened a prior therapist and had smashed his windshield, although the therapist took no action afterward. Dr. Senior was convinced that the snake delivery represented acting out in the transference, and that Ms. Troubled was not primarily interested in harming Dr. Victim.

Meanwhile, Ms. Troubled was still at large, her whereabouts unknown. Dr. Victim requested police protection, and they accompanied her home that evening and carefully searched the premises.

Dr. Victim spent the next 5 days frightened and angry, while she struggled unsuccessfully to obtain some assistance in protecting herself from Ms. Troubled. She spoke repeatedly with each of Ms. Troubled's current treating professionals. One stated that he did not believe she was a danger, doubted that she was committable, and refused initially to evaluate her for possible commitment. After Dr. Victim vigorously expressed her concerns to him, he reevaluated the patient. He again concluded the patient was not committable, and he told Dr. Victim he had fulfilled his obligations.

The second professional stated that he had no responsibility to do anything because he was only evaluating the patient, not treating her. He saw Ms. Troubled once after this episode and did not evaluate her for possible commitment. Later, she left a message on his answering machine terminating with him.

Dr. Victim promptly made a criminal complaint against Ms. Troubled—assault with a dangerous weapon, to wit, a snake. The local police were sympathetic but were slow to act. Initially, they had promised Dr. Victim that a warrant would be issued, but later they told her they would not issue a warrant but would instead issue a criminal complaint. This meant that Ms. Troubled would remain at large indefinitely. Dr. Victim had the clear impression that the police regarded this as a mental health matter rather than a police and criminal matter. They thought Ms. Troubled should be hospitalized.

The stalemate continued. Neither the police nor the mental health professionals were making any effort to apprehend Ms. Troubled. Dr. Victim then consulted an attorney and a forensic psychiatrist. Reviewing the history, the forensic psychiatrist was doubtful about the patient's committability. He urged Dr. Victim and her attorney to attend the clerk's hearing at which the court would decide how to deal with her complaint. Dr. Victim did so, and as a result of her vigorous advocacy, the court issued an arrest warrant. Six days after placing the snake in the box, Ms. Troubled was finally taken into custody. She was brought to court where she was evaluated for competency.

The court psychiatric evaluation found Ms. Troubled to be competent and not mentally ill within the meaning of the commitment statute. The judge who heard the facts was sufficiently persuaded of the defendant's possible danger to Dr. Victim that she set bail. The defendant could not meet the bail and was ordered to state prison to await trial.

A member of the prison mental health team met with Ms. Troubled while she was awaiting trial. Ms. Troubled told her that she was very angry at Dr. Senior for terminating. She related her fantasies of putting a snake in his mailbox, but decided to give it to Dr. Victim because "she would not know who it was from. I had no intention of hurting her. I just wanted to scare her and get attention. If I had given it to Dr. Senior I would not have been able to handle his anger and my anger. I could tolerate it better if it was someone I did not know."

She had telephoned her therapists immediately after delivering the snake because, she said, "I felt bad about it. There would be some reactions, restraining orders. So I called the therapists so they would stop it before it got to her." She reported all this in an even tone with little facial expression. She added, "The anger is still there. I know I would never hurt him. What I did was for attention."

Later, Ms. Troubled pleaded guilty. The judge placed her on probation with psychiatric treatment as a condition. On 1-year follow-up, she was in treatment with an experienced therapist. He reported that therapy was progressing well, and that she had an excellent job and had been given a promotion. There were no further episodes of antisocial or violent behavior.

Discussion

The case of Ms. Troubled illustrates the difficulties of doing intensive psychotherapy with patients who have poor ability to modulate affect. When strong affects are aroused in the transference, violence is possible. Except for the bizarre nature of the violent episode, this is a typical history for a woman with borderline personality disorder.

This case also illustrates that psychiatrists cannot predict violence accurately in the individual case. Dr. Senior was experienced; he knew his patient well and he had treated similar patients. Nevertheless, he failed to assess the potential for violence accurately.

Suppose Dr. Victim had picked up this package and had been bitten and seriously injured, an outcome she escaped in part by pure luck. Suppose she had died. Her survivors, having no personal relationships with the professionals involved, might sue. It would then be a legitimate question whether Dr. Victim had been damaged directly as a result of Dr. Senior's failure to assess his patient accurately, or as a result of the failure of either of the two current mental health professionals seeing her to warn of her peril.

Arguably, Dr. Senior was not liable, because the harm to Dr. Victim was not foreseeable at the time he terminated with Ms. Troubled. Nevertheless, his defense would depend to a great extent on how carefully he had evaluated Ms. Troubled for potential violence, and on how well he had documented his evaluation. Chapter 3 on private practice discusses in detail how that evaluation should be done.

In fact, Dr. Senior had obtained consultation from several senior colleagues. One thought Dr. Senior's concerns were pure countertransference, and he discounted them. Another thought there was no reason for concern, but that Dr. Senior's feelings had some validity.

Given this hypothetical scenario, the two current therapists might well be liable. Clearly, there was foreseeable harm when Ms. Troubled telephoned them. She told the professionals about a potentially lethal threat to Dr. Victim and initially neither of them responded. Fortunately, one of them eventually did, and Dr. Victim was not harmed.

Many mental health professionals would have responded as the two therapists did, avoiding involvement. They were frightened by the potential violence, and frightened by the potential legal involvement. Many professionals fear court involvement like the plague. This case, with elements of criminal conduct and potential civil liability, would frighten almost anyone.

In this case, the first therapist's judgment that the patient did not meet standards for civil commitment was supported by the judgment of the forensic psychiatrist. However, his initial refusal to become involved did not protect him and left Dr. Victim at continued risk.

The second therapist's belief that his limited involvement excused him from any further action is almost certainly erroneous. Had violence occurred, a court might well have found him to have been not merely negligent but grossly negligent.

The case illustrates with special clarity that patients often make these threats to therapists precisely because they expect therapists to respond by preventing the threatened violence, and Ms. Troubled later said she had done exactly that. In this case, the legal duty and the clinical responsibility converge on a single action—warning the victim.

The clinicians in this case could have done more than warn the victim. Optimally, Ms. Troubled's therapist should have engaged her in a discussion of the meaning of her action after she confessed what she had done. Exploring with this patient some of her rage and her reasons for its displacement might have helped her reality test whether her act would achieve her fantasied purpose. It would have been in Ms. Troubled's interest to take an active part in undoing her acting out. If the psychotherapist tried and failed to help the patient decide to undo her act, he should then have warned Dr. Victim or the receptionist.

Finally, the case illustrates the role of forensic psychiatry in the general practice of psychiatry. The forensic psychiatrist's knowledge of the courts and his clinical acumen were both essential to the eventual resolution of this case. When patients break the law, it is often in everyone's interest that charges be pressed. In this case, the protection of the victim and the ultimate constructive disposition for the patient both followed from the involvement of the court.

Concluding Remarks

The authors of this book have dealt with a wide variety of clinical situations that share the characteristic that the patient may do some foreseeable harm to another person. All these situations are fraught with conflicts that make it difficult for the therapist to act.

The first conflict is not so obvious but is important to recognize. On the one hand is the therapist's wish to be reflective, safe, untroubled, and secure in his or her office. On the other hand is the perceived need to take action when real danger threatens. Courage is rarely called for in the practice of psychiatry. But the case examples in this book illustrate clinical situations in which courage is called for. Sometimes it is moral courage—the courage to do something difficult even at some potential cost to oneself, such as reporting a colleague who has sexually abused a patient. Rarely, physical courage may be called for, as when the therapist fears that acting to protect the victim will turn the patient's anger toward the therapist. The mental health professional who files a child protective order may fear some retaliation from the parent who stands to have this child removed.

There is a danger that we as professionals displace our fear and our anger from the clinical dangers to hypothetical legal problems. We rail at the fact of potential liability and curse the plaintiffs' attorneys who have the power to make our lives miserable. Surely this misses the essential point. It is the clinical reality described in these chapters that is the source of almost all our difficulty and all our conflicts. These cases are distinguished by the fact that they rarely have easy solutions. Almost always, they involve a conflict between the need to maintain confidentiality and the need to protect someone. The clinician who maintains his or her clinical focus in the face of this foreseeable harm is most likely to protect society, the patient, and himself or herself.